A LIFE
Shaken

*My Encounter
with Parkinson's Disease*

Joel Havemann

FOREWORD BY STEPHEN G. REICH, M.D.

The Johns Hopkins University Press / Baltimore and London

Notes to the Reader

This book is not meant to substitute for medical care of people with Parkinson's disease, and treatment should not be based solely on its contents. Instead, treatment must be developed in a dialogue between the individual and his or her physician.

In view of ongoing research, changes in governmental regulations, and the constant flow of information relating to drug therapy and drug reactions, the reader is urged to check the package insert of each drug for any change in indications and dosage and for warnings and precautions.

The Johns Hopkins University Press
2715 North Charles Street
Baltimore, Maryland 21218–4363
www.press.jhu.edu

Library of Congress Cataloging-in-Publication Data
Havemann, Joel.
    A life shaken : my encounter with Parkinson's disease / Joel
Havemann ; foreword by Stephen G. Reich.
        p. cm.
Includes bibliographical references and index.
    ISBN 0-8018-6928-5 (hbk. : alk. paper)
    1. Havemann, Joel—Health. 2. Parkinson's
disease—Patients—United States—Biography. I. Title.
    RC382 .H385 2002
    362.1'96833'0092—dc21
2001004650

A catalog record for this book is available from the British Library.

To Judy,
who made it all happen

And to Anne, Margaret, and William,
who make it all worthwhile

Contents

Foreword

I HAVE HAD THE PRIVILEGE OF SERVING as Joel Havemann's neurologist since February 5, 1990. But his book has made me feel more like an obstetrician. I have seen it mature from conception, through early development, and, now, delivery. This book has two parents, both found in Joel, and each has contributed something unique. The first is a professional journalist who has written an objective, detailed, lucid account of Parkinson's disease—in my view, the best by a non-physician. The reader looking for accurate information on Parkinson's will find it here. The second parent is a middle-aged husband and father who, just as he seemed to have the world by the tail, had his grip loosened by Parkinson's disease. Joel's personally revealing account of living day-to-day, and year-to-year, with Parkinson's disease is the soul of this book. It is a story told vividly and passionately with all the highs and lows, fears, frustrations, insights, struggles, victories, and losses—big and small—faced by those with Parkinson's disease.

For Joel, as for all people with Parkinson's disease, the news of the diagnosis was tragic. He was truly *shaken*. And yet, while there is a background of tragedy in the pages that follow, this story can and should be viewed as a tale of heroism. When, as Joel relates, the simple act of flipping a pancake presents a challenge, it is easy to appreciate the perseverance and courage needed just to get up every day determined to live as normal a life as possible. Joel, like multitudes of others with Parkinson's, does so. And he, like others similarly affected, probably doesn't consider himself a hero. But doing the ordinary under extraordinary limitations is undeniably heroic.

Overly humble, Joel does not reveal in this book that he was one of several recipients of the first, and now annual, "Buddy Awards," presented at a fundraising gala for Parkinson's in 2000. This award, named after Barton "Buddy" Levenson, another remarkable patient of mine, embodies the determination, integrity, equanimity, and optimism he demonstrated in a long battle with Parkinson's disease.

Joel recounts the details from his first visit to me on February 5, 1990. I, too, despite seeing many patients, have a clear memory of that visit. Tall and thin (read on for his gentle account of my own, rather opposite, physiognomy), he impressed me with his background as a Harvard mathematics graduate and his current position as a senior editor with the *Los Angeles Times*. I could also tell he was scared to death—that "deer in the headlights" look that, after fifteen years of practice, I have never grown accustomed to and hope I never will. By the time a person with Parkinson's disease makes it to the trained eye of a Parkinson's specialist, the diagnosis is usually obvious in the waiting room. That's the easy part. The hard part is delivering the diagnosis. In the back of every new patient's mind is the hope that maybe the problem is a ruptured disk or nerves or benign essential tremor—anything but Parkinson's.

The diagnosis of Parkinson's disease, especially in young people like Joel, usually sets off a spiral of worst-case scenarios. No amount of reassurance on my part seems to help at this stage. But slowly, and remarkably, people with Parkinson's and their families learn that there is life after the diagnosis. Fortunately, the disease progresses slowly, and at least for the intermediate future, anti-parkinsonian medications do a pretty good job of controlling the symptoms.

Successful management of Parkinson's disease depends on more than just taking medications. On a daily basis, I have the privilege of observing people like Joel cope amazingly well. From them, I have developed an acronym that I hope will help readers with Parkinson's and those who care for someone with the disease: HOPE for coping. The *H* stands for honesty and humor. Honestly facing the diagnosis of Parkinson's and willingly sharing it with others are cornerstones of effective coping. Just after being diagnosed, Joel went so far as to have his situation posted on the computer bulletin board at work. This prevented rumors and, by demonstrating that the subject was not taboo, helped to avoid pity from co-workers. Not everyone is so forthcoming so quickly. Every person has to find the appropriate time to share the diagnosis with family, friends, and colleagues. After doing so, many patients have expressed their relief to me. Although there is nothing funny about Parkinson's, as you'll see in Joel's book, humor, the second characteristic of successful coping, can be a potent antidote, particularly when the alternative is crying—which is not a bad coping strategy, either, from time to time.

The *O* in HOPE stands for optimism. Viewing the glass as half-empty or half-full may be more innate than learned or cultivated, but successful coping with Parkinson's relies on emphasizing the small victories and de-emphasizing the defeats. For example, it would have been easy for Joel to bypass an opportunity to spend three years in Brussels reporting on the European economy, but he took the chance and his accomplishments overshadowed the tribulations of Parkinson's.

Perseverance is the *P* in HOPE and another quality I see in those who manage to cope well with the disease: they simply don't give up. When getting out of bed in the morning, putting toothpaste on the toothbrush, and getting dressed take extra time and effort, it would be much easier just to stay in bed. But successful copers persevere, determined to lead as normal a life as possible and view obstacles not as insurmountable but as challenges.

For the *E* in HOPE, I'm preaching to the converted. Readers of this book are already arming themselves with one of the most potent weapons in the battle against Parkinson's: education. Understanding the disease, the medications, and the latest research helps to provide a sense of control. I find it much easier and more productive to treat an educated patient; the doctor-patient relationship, so important for a chronic disease like Parkinson's, becomes one of teamwork rather than paternalism. You will find in these pages an up-to-date account of Parkinson's disease which strikes a perfect balance between enough sophistication to make it credible and meaningful and enough of the journalist's touch to make it readable and understandable.

Since 1989, when Joel first developed Parkinson's disease, tremendous advances have been made: no fewer than half a dozen new drugs; a renaissance in surgical therapy; the discovery of several genes causing Parkinson's; considerably more public and private funds available to fight Parkinson's; the growth and preeminence of the Parkinson's Study Group, a consortium of investigators in North America devoted to experimental therapeutics; new discoveries in the laboratory on the basic mechanisms underlying the death of dopamine nerve cells; and exciting leads about what causes Parkinson's. And this is just a partial list. As Joel's book poignantly demonstrates, and as other people struggling with Parkinson's know equally well, there is still a long way to go. But I am optimistic that it will not be long before this book, and others on Parkinson's, will be found in the history section of libraries and bookstores.

Stephen G. Reich, M.D.
Associate Professor, Neurology
The Johns Hopkins University School of Medicine
Director, Parkinson's Disease and Movement Disorders Center
The Johns Hopkins Medical Institutions

Acknowledgments

NO ONE WITH PARKINSON'S DISEASE can lead a fully independent life. As the symptoms accumulate, we depend more and more on others—family, friends, co-workers, others with Parkinson's, even sometimes strangers—to help us manage the routine tasks that slowly become unmanageable on our own. So it has been with this book. I couldn't have compiled these chapters without considerable help from the experts: the medical professionals, the Parkinson's community, and others. I thank them all.

At the beginning I had no idea how difficult it would be to learn, let alone explain, the way the brain works and the way the Parkinson's brain doesn't work. Helping me along the way were some of the best teachers in the land: Roy Bakay, Ted Dawson, Valina Dawson, Roger Duvoisin, Curt Freed, John Gearhart, Philip Gildenberg, Mark Hallett, Frederick Lenz, Ken Marek, Harold Mars, Ron McKay, Mihail Polymeropoulos, Ira Shoulson, Lisa Shulman, Joseph Steiner, and William Weiner. I owe a special debt to Fred Wooten, head of neurology at the University of Virginia, who helped me through some particularly rough spots, and to Elisabeth Leach, who linked us up.

Then there are the people with Parkinson's who generously shared their experiences with me: the activists, Perry Cohen, Jim Cordy, and Joan Samuelson; the politician, Janet Reno; and the many whose stories are so inspirational and instructive: Ed Calhoon, Tom Collins, Art Cook, Sandra Forney, Stephanie Fromer, Rusty Glazer, Barbara Gormly, Dana Gunnison, Stan Hamburger, Sam Joseloff, Nina King, Michael Kushnick, David Laventhol, Larry McCurdy, Lisa Mummert, Don Nelson, Leon Paparella, and Sandra Pollock. And a tip of the hat to Becky Dunlop, who set me up with many of the above.

In the category of caregivers, Parkinson's unsung heroes, I benefited from the experiences of Donna Dorros, Susan Hamburger, and Carolyn Nelson. A special thanks to Morton Kondracke, who wrote the book about caregiving (*Saving Milly*) and who helped me launch mine.

The *Los Angeles Times* gave me, no questions asked, the time I needed to complete the manuscript. Thanks in particular to Jack Nelson and Dick Cooper for giving me their encouragement and to Doyle

McManus and Tom McCarthy for putting up with my peculiar habits. Among the health journalists who shared their ideas and information with me were Marlene Cimons, Sheryl Stolberg, and Aaron Zitner.

Thanks to those who read all or parts of the manuscript and provided both encouragement and constructive criticism—not always an easy combination. Two Parkinson's patients, Rusty Glazer and David Laventhol (a former publisher of the *Los Angeles Times*), read passages and gave me boosts at crucial junctures. At the Johns Hopkins University Press, executive editor Jacqueline Wehmueller championed my cause and offered sound advice. Alice Porter, a dear friend, read a draft from start to finish and offered a particularly coherent critique. John Alexander, a good friend, gave me a historian's perspective. Bunli Yang, a friend indeed, not only provided editorial guidance but also, by being there when the going got rough, helped keep me going.

Finally, my special thanks to three who are in categories all their own.

Stephen G. Reich of the Johns Hopkins University played two essential roles. As Dr. Reich, he defied the maxim that neurologists don't care about their individual patients. His personal attention is responsible in no inconsiderable degree for the fact that I'm still active nearly twelve years after he diagnosed my Parkinson's. And as my friend Stephen, he read every chapter as I completed it and corrected misstatements and misinterpretations. If the book in the end is moderately optimistic about the outlook for those of us with Parkinson's disease, it's because he said countless times, "Well, it's your book, but I really don't think you have to be quite so downbeat."

Bob Samuelson managed to cement his position in my very small circle of close friends even while playing the indispensable role as exacting editor of the manuscript. He was able (could he have learned from his own Judy?) to find kind ways to say, "You call this a chapter? Where's the rest of it?" and, "You've got the information, but nobody will ever be able to tell that if you present it this way." No writer ever built up a greater debt to a colleague than I to him.

And finally there is my family: Ethel Ellersiek and Bruce Bohle, who shared their experiences with me and read and critiqued an entire draft of the manuscript; Theresa Nicol, Edward Herskovits, and little Evelyn, who taught me about small quantities of spices and small packages of joy; and of course, Judy and our children. Anne, Margaret, and William may never really know me other than shaky; I hope they also know me as strong. Judy made the book possible by leaving me lots of room and time to write. She read the manuscript from front to back at least twice and offered a valuable mix of editorial and spousal advice. But those comments trivialize her contribution. She is more than I could have asked of life, and I love her dearly.

A Life Shaken

Introduction: *As I Lay Trembling*

> The disease, respecting which the present inquiry is made, is of a nature
> highly afflictive. . . . The unhappy sufferer has considered it as an evil,
> from the domination of which he had no prospect of escape.
> —James Parkinson, *An Essay on the Shaking Palsy*

THIS DAY SHOULD BE PRIME TIME FOR ME. It's the first Monday in February 1997: President Bill Clinton is sending his annual budget to a hostile Congress. As a senior editor in the Washington bureau of the *Los Angeles Times,* I oversee the stories that our reporters are writing about Clinton's budget. At 6 P.M., three hours before the deadline for punching the computer button that sends our stories to Los Angeles, I should be coiled at my keyboard, honing the stories that will appear in more than a million newspapers in southern California tomorrow under a bold headline extending across most of the top of the front page.

Instead, I'm flat on my back on a couch that's too short in a windowless room in the bureau. I can't even sit at a computer, much less make a keyboard work. My arms and legs are shaking uncontrollably. Although I am only 53 years old, I have already been struggling with Parkinson's disease for seven years. And right now the disease is winning.

I take one of the tablets that are supposed to suppress the symptoms, hoping that this one will be more effective than the last. Then I stretch out, my head awkwardly perched on one arm of the couch. To restrain my shaking legs, I wedge my feet up against the opposite arm. Likewise, I tuck my arms under my back. Neither strategy works. The muscles in my legs and arms become rigid to the point of pain. I have to move them to release the pressure. Then they go right on shaking. I attempt to concentrate on something other than my body. It has to be something complicated enough to capture my attention without making me worry. I try counting by thirteens in French. *Treize,* I say to myself as I try to take a deep breath. *Vingt-six. Trente-neuf.* After five or ten minutes, this begins to help. At last, somewhere around 650 (13 added to itself 50 times), I begin to relax.

Then the switchboard operator announces on the office loudspeaker, "Telephone call for Joel Havemann. Joel, you have a phone call." I have no intention of taking the call. But just thinking about it upsets my delicate equilibrium. I have been balancing on the edge of an abyss. A tiny push throws me ever so slightly off balance. Slowly, gradually, I lean farther and farther into the abyss until, inevitably, I come crashing down. I am shaking worse than before.

Six hundred sixty-three.... Six hundred seventy-six.... Six hundred eighty-nine.

How much longer can I go on like this? How much longer will the Los Angeles Times pay me if, at any moment, my brain can lose control of my body? In the windowless room, unwelcome images dance across my brain. "Why me?" I wonder. Out in the newsroom, on the other side of the closed door, several dozen others work in my office, many of them older than I. Not one of them has Parkinson's—or any other degenerative disease, for that matter. What have I done that has landed me on this side of the door? Not a thing, I'm sure. There is no grand plan. All is chance. I'm lucky to be an American, lucky to have a wonderful family and a great job—and unlucky to have Parkinson's. That doesn't make me feel any better. It's just the way it is.

As it happens, earlier today the Associated Press sent its client newspapers a story about a promising new treatment for Parkinson's, involving the introduction of a particular gene into the brains of rats with Parkinson's disease. Next the researchers plan to try their gene on African green monkeys; if that works, humans will follow. But the very last sentence of the Associated Press story issues a familiar caution: "If the therapy works with primates, it could be ready for human tests in five to ten years."

Five to ten years? How often have I heard that before? It has been exactly one day longer than seven years since I was diagnosed with Parkinson's disease. During that time, countless medical researchers have held out the promise of new treatments for Parkinson's within five to ten years. In my seven years and a day, nothing that I regard as a major advance has occurred. In my early Parkinson's years, I confidently figured my timing was just about right: I could manage well enough with the disease until medical science discovered something new to subdue it. But now I wonder. From where I lie, medical science scarcely seems to be making progress. Society is spending zillions to combat cancer and AIDS—and, by comparison, hardly anything on Parkinson's. But cancer and AIDS kill; Parkinson's mostly cripples. So what? Cancer and AIDS are them. Parkinson's is me.

Nine hundred eighty-eight. One thousand one. One thousand fourteen.

Why am I feeling sorry for myself? At least I wasn't born a generation earlier. Until the late 1960s, the standard treatment for Parkinson's was almost entirely ineffective. Only then did researchers develop a drug that (more or less) substitutes for the chemical whose absence from the brain causes Parkinson's. If I had been born when my father was, I probably would have spent all of every day either shaking uncontrollably or so sedated that I couldn't even shake. As it is, for most of every day I don't look much different from everyone on the other side of the closed door. When my pills are working, I can move as smoothly as the next guy. I can live life pretty much as I did before Parkinson's landed me in the windowless room.

And there's plenty to live for. The *Los Angeles Times* actually pays me to do what I enjoy doing anyway—learning about interesting things and writing about them. More than that, much more, I have a family better than any man deserves. Judy, my wife, has given me so much—including our three children. I can scarcely remember what life was like without Anne, who is now 15, and Margaret and William, 11-year-old twins. Nor do I particularly care to. Life with them is (usually) sweet.

One thousand one hundred thirty-one. One thousand one hundred forty-four. One thousand one hundred fifty-seven.

But despite my best efforts, bleak images drive out the cheery in the darkness of the windowless room. Thoughts of family turn to my father, Ernest. He lived with us for the last two years of his life, the last six months as an invalid with a mind that kept on working but a body that gave up. He died in my arms one lovely June morning two years ago because he no longer had the strength to breathe through the phlegm in his pneumonia-ridden lungs. Now my mother-in-law is about to take Dad's place in our household. Lola McIntosh's tiny body is as strong as steel; it is her mind that has forsaken her. Sometimes she recognizes Judy, my wife, as her daughter; sometimes she thinks Judy is her mother. I'm almost always a total stranger, and she thinks of her grandchildren as "that boy" and "those girls." A failed body, a failed mind. Is that what my own illness might ultimately visit on me?

I can't stop thinking the unthinkable: About Mo Udall, who was diagnosed with Parkinson's in 1978, two years after finishing second to Jimmy Carter in the race for the Democratic presidential nomination. Although he managed to serve in the U.S. Congress for twelve more years, he has lain in a "rest home" for the past six years, comatose from a head injury incurred when he lost his balance and fell down the stairs of his home. (He died in the rest home in 1998.) . . . About surgeons unable to perform what seems in 1997 to be one of the most promising operations for Parkinson's—replacing diseased brain cells with healthy ones from fetuses. The government has all but stopped paying for research using tissue from aborted fetuses. . . . About the crushing burden that will fall on Judy if I become completely incapacitated. . . . About the prospect that our children will have no memories of me before I had the "shaky disease."

One thousand three hundred ninety-one. One thousand four hundred four. One thousand four hundred seventeen.

Finally, about half an hour after taking my last pill, I feel my arms and legs relax. Exhausted, I close my eyes and drift off to sleep. Soon I awaken, my arms and legs as steady as they were twenty years ago. With Parkinson's, it feels so good just to feel ordinary. I bolt from the couch. The deadline is approaching. There are stories to edit.

This is a story of Parkinson's disease: of what the disease does to the 500,000 to 1.5 million Americans (and countless more millions around the world) who have it; of what we can do to treat it today, of what we might be able to do tomorrow. The disease that sent me fleeing to the windowless room that February afternoon remains at its core a mystery, even though medical science knows more about it than almost any other neurological disorder. Nearly two hundred years have elapsed since James Parkinson, a London physician who gained fame initially as an analyst of animal and plant fossils, recognized the disease in three of his own patients and three others whom he observed at a distance. All six exhibited the same symptoms: tremor, stooped posture, and generally slow movements. But Parkinson had no idea what caused the symptoms. Only in the late 1950s did researchers identify a brain chemical called dopamine and discover that damage to the part of the brain that manufactures dopamine was a common feature of people with Parkinson's. Even today, the disease continues to taunt us. Just when we think it attacks one part of the brain, we learn that it has other targets as well. Just when we conclude that it cannot be hereditary—how else to explain why Parkinson's frequently strikes one identical twin but not the other?—scientists identify the precise genetic villain in some families in which Parkinson's is common.

That Parkinson's should be mysterious is no mystery. It's a disease of the human brain, the most complex three-pound object on earth. So intricate is the brain's chemical circuitry that, by comparison, the typical desktop computer of the mid-1990s had the problem-solving capacity of a snail.[1] And the brain is more, much more, than an unimaginably powerful computer. Only the human brain is capable of emotion; only the human brain can achieve "consciousness." Computers, like people, can plan brilliant chess strategy. But only people can feel elated about winning and devastated about losing; only people can reflect upon how satisfying it would feel to win and how upsetting to lose. The wonder is not that things in the brain go wrong from time to time—that people suffer from Parkinson's and Alzheimer's, from schizophrenia and depression, and from all the other illnesses that can be traced to glitches in the brain's extraordinary circuitry. The wonder is that, for the most part, the brain functions flawlessly for as long as a hundred years and more. Computers crash all the time—the system at my local motor vehicles department seems to be down more than it's up. An organ as complex as the brain but as reliable as a computer would never be up.

Just as Parkinson's is one of the best understood neurological diseases, so is it among the most effectively treated. But that has been true for only a short while. For a century and a half after Parkinson, the disease bearing his name defied not only those who tried to cure it but even those who sought merely to alleviate its symptoms. Those unfortunates who contracted Parkinson's disease before the late 1960s faced a future of slowly building agony as their brains lost control of their bodies. Now there is a welcome variety of medications (I take five before breakfast) and surgical techniques to make the brain do what it's supposed to do, or at least not do what it isn't supposed to. As a result, people like me can look forward to many good years while the disease is in its early stages. That fact, ironically, may work to our ultimate disadvantage. Most of us who can manage okay with Parkinson's (and I put myself firmly in this camp) put up a bold public front for as long as we can and behave as if we were perfectly normal, despite the dread of the future that we all harbor inside. All of us with the disease would probably be better off if more of us were to stand up in public and demand that medical science do more not just to treat this scourge but to cure it.

In the chapters that follow, the story of Parkinson's is tightly intertwined with my very personal adventure with it. For an adventure it is— not one that I would have chosen, but an adventure all the same. Parkinson's pushed me over my own personal Rubicon. Even if medical science finds a cure in time for me (an increasingly unlikely prospect), I will never be the person I was before. The disease has forced me to learn things about myself that I had been able to ignore. It has left me face to face with some of life's imponderables: Why are we here? What in life is important, what is trivial? What should we accomplish before we die?

In the pages that follow I will seek to provide my own answers—as much for my own edification as for the reader's. Perhaps because I am a writer by trade, I am confronting Parkinson's by committing some of my innermost thoughts to print.

I trust I am not so arrogant as to believe my life's code should guide others. The world is already overrun with those who would force their views on others. At the same time, I hope my experience will prove of some small value not only to those who have Parkinson's disease or love someone who does but also to the millions who suffer from other degenerative diseases. Only in the century just ended have people in large numbers had to struggle with long-term diseases. Until then, they simply didn't live long enough. Half of all Americans who were born in 1850 died before their fortieth birthday; for those born in 1900, fewer than half made it to age 50. Thanks to modern techniques of public health, Americans who are born today can figure to live well into their 70s. That leaves plenty of time for parts of the body to wear out or succumb to attack by outside agents.

All of us have our individual ways of coping with a future in which each tomorrow will find us a little sicker than we are today. Particularly useful, I have found, is not taking life in general or oneself in particular too seriously. *Homo sapiens* has inhabited this planet for many thousands of years, and our descendants will probably be around for many thousands more. Our species has come a long way since our ancestors climbed down from the trees, where their forebears had lived, and learned to walk on two feet, freeing up their hands to perform such valuable tasks as making tools, cultivating the land, and typing books on computer keyboards. In that vast expanse of time, it's difficult to imagine that anything that any of us does individually will make a whole lot of lasting difference. Percy Bysshe Shelley said it best two hundred years ago in his poem "Ozymandias," about the great monuments, now reduced to rubble, of a fictional king of ancient Egypt:

> And on the pedestal these words appear—
> "My name is Ozymandias, king of kings:
> Look on my works, ye Mighty, and despair!"
> Nothing beside remains. Round the decay
> Of that colossal wreck, boundless and bare
> The lone and level sands stretch far away.

CHAPTER ONE

Denial and Ignorance

> So slight and nearly imperceptible are the first inroads of this malady, and so extremely slow its progress, that it rarely happens, that the patient can form any recollection of the precise period of its commencement. The first symptoms perceived are, a slight sense of weakness, with a proneness to trembling in some particular part, sometimes in the head, but most commonly in one of the hands and arms.
>
> —James Parkinson, *An Essay on the Shaking Palsy*

ALL OF US WITH PARKINSON'S DISEASE have a story to tell about how we found out. The story, like the disease itself, often unfolds slowly and takes some surprising twists. Parkinson's does not announce itself with a dramatic and debilitating attack but rather with a long series of minor jabs at our self-control. Even when the warning signs are undeniable, we try to deny them—in part because the disease is so far out of the public consciousness, in part because we naturally reject the prospect of living out the rest of our lives with a degenerative disease. I know all this now, but a decade ago I did not. My Parkinson's story starts with raspberries.

My boss and I were interviewing a job candidate over lunch early in 1989 in one of Washington's expense-account restaurants, the kind that are so overpriced that nobody would eat there unless somebody else were paying. For dessert I ordered raspberries (they must have cost about 25 cents a berry), only to discover that I couldn't get them from the bowl to my mouth with a spoon. My hand was too shaky; they kept falling off. I didn't think much of it. My hands had always been unsteady, a characteristic that I shared with my mother and had probably inherited from her.

It was only a few months, however, before my family and friends began to notice that my shakiness was becoming more pronounced. Mostly they didn't say anything; I assume they were too embarrassed, or thought I would be. My children had no such inhibitions. At the time, Margaret and William were only 3 years old, but Anne was just turning 7, old enough to notice how I was changing. "Daddy, you're shaking a lot," she told me more than once.

How come? My own father, who had an opinion on almost everything, figured it was stress. That made a certain amount of sense: If stress could make you shake, I was a good candidate. Life at home, though happy, was pressure-packed. Nine people squeezed into our little suburban house. Five of us—Judy, our three children, and I— occupied the three bedrooms on the second floor, with only Anne enjoying a room of her own. Judy's 25-year-old daughter and her boyfriend held down the attic, which consisted of a finished bedroom and living room but no bathroom. A small but complete apartment in the basement, where the garage used to be, was barely big enough for our live-in baby-sitter and her 5-year-old daughter.

This many bodies crammed into a small space is a formula for chaos, and mornings, when most people are naturally cranky, were particularly turbulent. As it happens, Judy is a fitful sleeper; more often than not she gets her best sleep just before dawn. So responsibility for seeing that everybody was fed and out of the house fell largely to me. Frequently I was exhausted by the time I arrived at work.

Nor was it easy to relax there. The *Los Angeles Times* has more than thirty reporters in Washington who write about everyone from the president to the government's bureaucrats. To ride herd on this team of reporters, the *Times* also has six editors—one boss and five subordinates. I was one of the five; being older and more experienced than the others, I was generally regarded as the first among equals. Whenever my boss was missing from the action, I was more or less in charge. And in the late 1980s, he was often missing.

Had my home and professional lives conspired to give me the jitters? This seemed reasonable. What could I do about it? I didn't know; so I saw a doctor.

"I'm not sure medical science has a cure for what ails me," I told my family doctor in April of 1989. "But I don't know where else to start." The doctor, a big, bearded, affable fellow a few years younger than I, listened attentively but had no better idea than I did. He ran a bunch of routine tests, found nothing very significant, and sent me off to a neurologist downtown, where many of Washington's high-priced doctors cater to many of its high-paid lawyers and lobbyists.

Dr. DC's office, full of self-important receptionists and clerks and accountants, made you feel that he was doing you a huge favor just by agreeing to see you: that you were imposing on him merely by showing up. Well past my appointment time, one of the functionaries ushered me into the doctor's inner office, which was bristling with framed diplomas and documents certifying that he had completed this or that postgradu-ate training. Eyeing me with total assurance, he observed that my right leg and sometimes my right hand trembled when at rest. He tested my muscles and joints for stiffness and rigidity. He checked my hand-eye coordination and my reflexes. Finally, he ordered up an MRI of my brain—an extremely sophisticated (and expensive) scan that, in effect, slices the brain into cross sections and shows what's going on in each. After the MRI, I went back to Dr. DC for another consultation.

"Well, at least it doesn't look like you have Parkinson's," he said offhandedly. "I suspect you've been wondering about that, haven't you?" I admitted that the possibility had crossed my mind, although neither of us had mentioned it. But the MRI, Dr. DC said, showed no destruction of the nerve cells in the part of the brain whose decay unleashes Parkinson's symptoms. In addition, he said, my tremor was largely confined to my right arm and leg, and Parkinson's generally involves both sides of the body, not just one. The clincher was this: Hardly anybody comes down with Parkinson's at my young age of 45.

Only later did I learn that he had been mistaken on all counts. Even an MRI lacks the necessary power to reveal the destruction of nerve cells in the Parkinson's brain. The Parkinson's tremor generally begins on one side of the body and only gradually consumes the other side as well. And while few people develop Parkinson's as young as 45, it is by no means unknown even among people much younger. But at the time I knew none of this, and I was only too eager to believe the good news.

If it wasn't Parkinson's, what was it? Dr. DC concluded that I had a much-exaggerated version of the tremor that I had displayed all my life, the one I had presumably inherited from my mother. The medical phrase for it is familial tremor, although it is more commonly known as essential tremor. "You're not the first patient of mine whose essential tremor has suddenly grown worse," Dr. DC said. "I've been seeing a woman who's about your age, and she's going through the same thing." I've always wondered whether Dr. DC was wrong about her too.

Before he let me go, Dr. DC suggested two forms of treatment. For the next six months he put me on Inderal, a drug that is supposed to reduce essential tremor. It may have made me less shaky, but that is not all it did. "It completely changed your disposition," Judy said later. "Ordinarily you're just about the most easygoing, even-tempered per-son I know. During those six months you were in a terrible humor, you were cranky, you were grouchy, and even the children couldn't stand to be around you." It was in the middle of one summer night during this period that I tried to empty the bedroom dehumidifier, only to stumble in the dark and spill several quarts of water on the rug. "God damn son of a bitch," I stormed as I mopped up the damage, venting my frustrations and oblivious to Judy's silent wish that I shut up.

Dr. DC's second treatment was more fun for me and everyone around me: a tall glass of wine in the evening. Not being much of a drinker, I can't remember what effects that had on my tremor. But unlike the Inderal, it made me feel a lot better. Too bad the doctor couldn't prescribe it; that way, my health insurance would have paid for it. Wouldn't it be great to hand a pharmacist a prescription for a case of Chateau Lafite Rothschild?

Despite the Inderal and the wine, my shakiness gradually got worse. On cold nights, when I walked the two blocks from my office to the subway, I couldn't keep my right hand in my pocket the whole way because my arm would get too stiff. In November, I was supposed to carve the turkey for Anne's second-grade Thanksgiving celebration. Instead of slices, my unsteady hand hacked the turkey into rough chunks. "Why are you shaking so much?" one of Anne's classmates called out. "Because I enjoy it," I muttered under my breath. Another parent who was there said to Judy later, "Joel looked terrible. What's the matter?"

That sent me back to my family doctor, who was as baffled as he had been six months earlier. So this time, instead of a neurologist, he referred me to a biofeedback specialist. The result was one of life's more bizarre hours.

Biofeedback, I discovered, is a fancy name for a kind of relaxation therapy, a means of asserting voluntary control over what is ordinarily the involuntary nervous system—a high-tech form of self-hypnosis. Well, maybe more like mid-tech. My therapist, a matter-of-fact, not-too-friendly woman in her early 40s, sat me down in a big, brown-leather lounge chair and, for thirty minutes, interviewed me about my complaints. "I've had a tremor in my right arm and right leg for the better part of two years," I said. "It seems to get worse with stress. Dr. DC has diagnosed it as essential tremor." As an afterthought I added something I hadn't planned to say at all: "But I don't really believe it."

"Why not?" she wanted to know.

"Because it keeps getting worse."

"Then what do you think it is?"

"I wish I knew. Stress? My bad back? Can these things make you shake?"

Stress, she said, could certainly aggravate a tremor, if not cause it. So she asked me about my daily routine: coping with my three small children at home, trying to manage a high-pressure job.

"What do you do for lunch when you're working?" she asked.

"Usually I just eat a couple of sandwiches at my desk. I don't have time to do much more."

"You mean you don't take the time," she corrected me. "Everybody needs to have a little down time during the day. Even if you don't go out to a restaurant, try to have your sandwiches away from your desk and away from the telephone."

Sound advice, I'm sure. But I got home late enough as it was; if I indulged myself in a leisurely lunch hour, I wasn't sure I'd ever get home in time to see my children while they were still awake.

After thirty minutes of chitchat, my therapist summoned the tools of her trade. To the palm of my left hand she taped a small gizmo that measured clamminess—a clammy hand being a sign of agitation. To my forehead she taped three electrodes that were wired to a small device that made a tone, something like the chime of a clock, every second or so.

"The more nervous you are, the higher the tone will be," she explained. "As you relax, the tone will grow lower, until, when you're perfectly calm, the tone will disappear. You'll find that you'll be able to put under voluntary control some body processes that are usually involuntary."

I wasn't entirely convinced, but I'd come this far and there was no turning back. She instructed me to push back on the arms of the lounge chair until the back tilted backward and the bottom part of the front of the chair converted into a footrest—only for my long legs it was more like a calf-rest, with my feet dangling uncomfortably off the end. The tone machine started making very-high-frequency sounds.

"Just lie back comfortably and close your eyes," she said quietly. "Close your eyes and take deep, comfortable breaths." Sure enough, the chimes from the tone machine came down in pitch. "You can feel the pressure flowing out of your scalp and your forehead. You can feel the muscles smoothing out. . . .

"Now focus your mind on your eyes. Your eyelids are heavy. Just let them lie there. Your eyes are getting heavy too. You can even feel the backs of your eyes as gravity holds them down. . . .

"Now concentrate on your jaw. Let gravity pull it down. Let gravity pull it down so that your mouth opens ever so slightly. Just let your jaw get heavy." To my astonishment, the chime machine stopped chiming. But not for very long.

"Now think about your arms," she instructed—and as I did, my right hand began its familiar tremor. The dreaded chime machine started chiming again at an ever-higher pitch. "Think about your arms," she repeated. (I am *already*, I thought to myself. That's the whole problem.) "Your arms are growing heavier. They are so heavy you can't lift them off the chair. Just let them rest there as you feel the tension flow out of them. Just let them rest there as the tension flows down your arms to your fingertips and out of your body." (The tone started coming back down again.) "The muscles of your arm are smooth and quiet and relaxed. Smooth and quiet and relaxed." (The chime machine went silent.)

Skipping a few parts of my anatomy, she ultimately arrived at my feet. "Let your toes relax and be heavy," she said in her slow, reassuring way. "The muscles in your toes are becoming smooth. You can feel the tension running out of your whole body through your toes."

Just when I was feeling mellow and celebrating the silence of the chime machine, the therapist turned the lights up and unhooked my electrodes. (She didn't have to detach the temperature sensor that she had taped to my left palm; it had worked loose during the session, even though my left hand was my steady one.) For a first-timer, she said, I had responded well. But before I committed to extended therapy, she suggested that I check in with my neurologist again to reassure myself that the cause of my jitters was stress, not something more serious and more difficult to reach with biofeedback.

So back to Dr. DC I went, demonstrably shakier than I had been when I had last seen him six months earlier. He had to admit that something actually seemed to be wrong with me. At one point in the examination, as I lay on my back, my arms and legs wouldn't rest comfortably. Instead, they bounced up and down like popcorn on a hot stove. "Wow," Dr. DC said, "you're shaking like anything."

No shit, Sherlock, I thought. I didn't need him to tell me that. My 7-year-old daughter already had. I needed him to explain why.

As a diagnostic test, he gave me a medication that moderates the tremor of Parkinson's disease. I was to come back in three weeks. After just a few days, the tremor had clearly diminished. Still, I stayed in denial. Rather than admit the obvious, I wove an elaborate theory that the tremor had something to do with the lower back spasms I'd had recently. Pinched nerves, I theorized, must account for my growing lack of body control.

It was then that my stepdaughter the medical student stepped in. "You need a doctor who knows what he's doing," Theresa told me. Before my next appointment with Dr. DC, she arranged for me to see a neurologist at the Johns Hopkins Hospital who specialized in diagnosing Parkinson's in young people. Judy, guessing what the outcome might be, came along on the one-hour drive to Baltimore.

There to greet us was Dr. Stephen G. Reich. Built solid and low to the ground like a Mercedes or a BMW, he seemed at first serious and even severe. With one of those pointy World War I helmets, he would have made a fine Prussian general. But he pronounced his name like *rich*, not like the Third *Reich*, and while his rich baritone was a tad formidable, his manner was sensitive and friendly.

It took him little more than one look to conclude that I had Parkinson's. But he didn't let on. Prudently, he examined me much as Dr. DC had. When I walked, my left arm swung naturally, but my right arm hung motionless. When I sat and rested my hands on my lap, my right hand began to shake. Apparently I was such a good specimen that Dr. Reich called in a colleague to have a look.

"Rest tremor . . . ," Dr. Reich whispered. "Classic pill-rolling." I felt cornered. No longer could I hide from what was ailing me. I had to face the dreaded word: *Parkinson's*. The date was February 5, 1990.

Dr. Reich tried to reassure me. "It's not the end of life as you know it," he said. "Parkinson's is like diabetes: it can be managed well even if it can't be cured." He told me that a new medication, only recently approved by federal drug regulators, held out considerable promise of retarding the disease. "If you take care of yourself," he said, "you could be good for many more years."

"But what will I be like when I'm 60?" I stammered.

"That," conceded Dr. Reich, "is impossible to predict."

I don't remember much of what happened for an hour or two after that. Judy says I was so upset that I let her drive home, something I did only under great duress. During the hour-long drive, Judy recalls, we chatted about this and that—about almost anything except what was really on our minds. Back home, we told the children as casually as we could that I had the "shaky disease." I didn't expect them to be alarmed. When I was about their age, my mother developed a disease called erysipelas, a quite painful infection of the skin that made her face swell up and her eyes nearly close. Far from worrying, I said she looked like a "Chinese bum." (Those were the days before political correctness.) I hoped my children would regard my disease equally as seriously. They didn't let me down. To this day, they think of me as shaky just as naturally as they think of me as tall. One recent spring day I was lying flat on my back on the deck behind our house, helping Anne study for her high school physics final even as I was trying to get my shaking under control. A few days later she remembered my helping her prepare for the test—but she had no memory of my condition.

More than a few Parkinson's patients try to keep their diagnosis a secret. Not me: too many people had already seen me shake, and I wanted them to know there was a good explanation. So I called Jack Nelson, who as chief of the *Los Angeles Times* Washington bureau was my boss's boss, and asked him to put the news of my diagnosis on the office's computer message system, with an appeal to my colleagues not to make a big fuss about it. Then I called two of my closest and oldest friends so that they wouldn't hear the news from some other source. Finally I called my parents, who lived in northern New Jersey but who that day were pursuing one of my dad's great passions: playing black-jack at the Atlantic City casinos. They seemed no more alarmed than my children. "You're not really surprised, are you?" Dad said. "Just about every other possibility had been ruled out." That made perfect sense. But somehow it didn't make me feel any better.

Next I went to the local library to read what I could find about Parkinson's. That made me feel even worse. In starkly clinical terms, the first medical reference books that I stumbled upon described a disease that was occasioned by the mysterious death of the cells in an obscure part of the brain buried deep under the huge lobes of nerve cells that enable us to think. The symptoms progressed inexorably from mild tremor and rigidity (that was me) to serious movement disorders— stooped posture, a shuffling gait, loss of balance, and a tendency to fall down. Impotence frequently waited along the Parkinson's road; so did incontinence. A little further along lurked dementia, and the all-but-inevitable destination was premature death.[1] That was a lot more than I could handle. I slammed those medical books shut and didn't open another for a very long time.

When I did, I discovered how remarkably little was known about Parkinson's disease: no wonder Dr. DC had difficulty diagnosing it. In 1817, when James Parkinson identified the disease, doctors were still applying leeches to the skin to suck out bad blood; in fact, Parkinson

himself claimed that leeches applied to the vertebrae in the neck con-
stituted one of the few effective treatments of the shaking palsy.[2] In
general, medicine couldn't do much for the injured and diseased. Eighteen years after Parkinson's groundbreaking monograph, Jacob Bigelow
of Harvard, then one of America's most eminent physicians, said it was
"the unbiased opinion of most medical men of sound judgment and
long experience" that "the amount of death and disaster in the world
would be less if all disease were left to itself."[3]

Surely the disease had existed long before Parkinson's name became
attached to it, although there is precious little evidence. Parkinson's is
predominantly a disease of the elderly, and until the twentieth century,
most people died of something else before being afflicted with Parkinson's. But there were some apparent exceptions. In a seventeenth-
century etching called the *Good Samaritan*, Rembrandt depicted a
stooped innkeeper whose outstretched hand seems to be shaking in the
familiar Parkinson's way. Galen, a Greek physician of the second century, wrote of patients whose hands trembled while at rest on their
laps—a telltale sign of Parkinson's. About 500 B.C., a Chinese medical
book referred to a disease characterized by limbs that shook "like the
leaves of a tree," and even before that, an Indian text described a disorder involving tremor, stiffness, and depression.[4] In fact, researchers in
San Jose, California, have found that Parkinson's disease can occur
naturally in squirrel monkeys. If at least a predisposition to getting the
disease is inherited through a faulty gene—and the evidence is increasingly pointing in this direction—then the disease must be at least as
old as the common ancestor of squirrel monkeys and *Homo sapiens*: six
or seven million years!

Slow as progress toward conquering the disease now seems to those
of us for whom every week matters, it was a whole lot slower in the
decades following Parkinson's monograph. Only in the 1860s did doctors first administer drugs that actually did Parkinson's patients any
good. Jean-Martin Charcot, a renowned Parisian neurologist, gave some
relief to some patients with a drug closely related to belladonna (literally,
"beautiful lady"), a plant whose extract was used to dilate the pupils of
Parisian showgirls to make them look more fetching. Doctors noticed
that belladonna also seemed to cause dry mouth, and so they used it on
Parkinson's patients to control drooling. That led quickly to the discovery that belladonna controls tremor. For many decades, belladonna
remained not only the best but also the only Parkinson's treatment.
Researchers were handicapped by not knowing where to look for the

central source of Parkinson's symptoms. Parkinson himself, admitting that he could do little more than guess, fingered the medulla oblongata, where the brain narrows down into the spinal cord. L. Ordenstein, a student of Charcot who analyzed thirty of Charcot's patients, noted in one a softening of the substantia nigra, a small, black mass of nerve cells somewhat higher up in the brain.[5] But it was not until the next century that his suspicion was confirmed; meanwhile, researchers wandered off in other directions.[6]

Nobody had a clue about what caused the disease, and some of the early theories seem laughable today. Charcot, suspecting sudden anxiety, told of a soldier's wife who contracted the disease when her husband's horse returned, riderless, from a civil disturbance in 1832. "Of the female patients whom we have interrogated," Charcot said, "many related how their complaint took its rise in the midst of the political commotion by which our country has been agitated."[7] This view persisted through the end of the century; New York physician Frederick Peterson recounted the case of an illicit whiskey distiller who came down with Parkinson's symptoms soon after the police discovered him.[8] Another popular suspect was prolonged exposure to cold, particularly damp cold. Ordenstein cited the case of a German man who developed Parkinson's soon after being attacked by Cossacks during the Napoleonic wars: the Cossacks stripped him of his clothes and forced him to lie down, covered with sweat, on the cold ground.[9] Gowers, one of the leading nineteenth-century British neurologists, wrote of the intriguing case of a 37-year-old woman who was sitting in a chair and minding her own business when a stream of water from a nearby tap unexpectedly flowed over her left wrist. Her left arm began trembling and never stopped, and the tremor spread gradually to her left leg and then to her right arm and leg.[10]

In the past four decades, medical science has made stupendous advances. A small blue pill, taken six times a day, is enough to keep me a productive member of society. For all the progress, however, the fundamental riddles of Parkinson's disease remain unsolved.

What are its symptoms? Most people who are diagnosed with Parkinson's start with most or all of the four cardinal symptoms: tremor of the arms and legs, stiffness of the arm and leg muscles, slowness of movement, and postural instability. But some have none of these symptoms or only one or two of them. A friend of mine with the same disease shares none of my symptoms; instead, he walks with a pronounced shuffle and frequently loses his balance. Many early symptoms are more bothersome than crippling: I frequently broke into a drenching sweat for no apparent reason, and I had trouble swallowing. Parkinson's also visited many of its common postural changes on me: I regularly found myself tilting far to the right while I sat, and occasionally I leaned so far forward while walking that I had to run to prevent myself from falling. The disease's progress varies as much as its initial symptoms. I'm one of the lucky ones: at seven years from my diagnosis as I write this passage, I can still type this sentence as accurately as I could have when I was 25, provided that I take my medication properly. Some who were diagnosed more recently than I are already totally disabled.

How many people have it? This question cannot be answered with any confidence as long as the diagnosis of Parkinson's is so uncertain. Besides, there is no central place that collects data from around the country. Consequently, estimates of the number of Americans with the disease range from half a million to one and a half million. Your estimate depends on your point of view. Those who are seeking more money to combat the disease are partial to the higher figure, while the medical profession leans toward the lower. It seems to me that an increasing proportion of new Parkinson's patients are younger than 50, as I was. But this is probably because it is the young patients, with much of their lives still ahead of them, who make the most noise demanding more work on a cure. Experts with a wider range of experience than I say that about 5 percent of all people with Parkinson's feel their first symptoms before the age of 40 and that the median age of onset is about 60, statistics that have been constant for many years. The disease strikes whites more commonly than other racial groups. It seems to favor males: about three men for every two women. The telltale signs of a Parkinson's brain are found in about 5 percent of people who are over 40 when they die and 10 percent of those who are over 70—even if they never displayed any Parkinson's symptoms. This suggests that for everyone with Parkinson's, another ten to twenty persons are on their way to having the disease but die first.[11]

What kinds of people get it? Interestingly, there is some evidence for a "Parkinson's personality"—a collection of traits that are more common among people with Parkinson's than in the rest of the population. We are said to be more cautious and less novelty seeking than others, characteristics that some researchers have linked to the same brain-chemical deficit that causes the tremor. Adjectives applied to us as a group include *industrious, rigid, moral, loyal, stoic, serious, frugal, orderly, persistent,* and *quiet.* We are also less likely to smoke than the non-Parkinson's population.[12] Ordinarily I put little stock in these kinds of generalizations about personality and behavior. But in this case, I have to admit that just about all the descriptions of the Parkinson's personality (except *rigid*) apply to me. And I haven't smoked a cigarette in my life. You have to be careful not to get causes and effects mixed up. It's not as if you could fend off Parkinson's by taking up smoking and mountain climbing and leaving your spouse. Rather, if you're already inclined in these directions, you're not so likely to develop Parkinson's.

What causes it? Researchers today are pretty confident that the culprits pointed to early on, including anxiety and exposure to the cold, were bogus. But some of the more recent hypotheses were just as goofy. In the first half of the twentieth century, one school of thought held that Parkinson's was a byproduct of the encephalitis epidemic that broke out worldwide after World War I. As many as 40 percent of the epidemic's survivors (including Adolf Hitler) developed Parkinson's, and if this had been the sole cause of the disease—as some researchers believed— it should have disappeared after the last of the encephalitis survivors died out, around 1980.[13] Obviously, this hypothesis turned out to be emphatically incorrect. To this day, researchers are still arguing over whether the cause is hereditary or environmental—or a combination. Environmental suspects have ranged from well water to a species of berry that grows on one half of the island of Guam, although the fact that Parkinson's can be found the world over suggests that any environmental toxins must be extremely common and widespread. Exponents of heredity gained ground in 1997 when scientists isolated a single defective gene in all the scores of members of an extended Italian and Italian-American family who have Parkinson's. However, researchers have since found this same bad gene in only a handful of other Parkinson's patients. And don't forget the many sets of identical twins in which only one twin has the disease.[14] Parkinson's probably results from some combination of heredity and environment—an inherited predisposition to contract the disease mixed with exposure to something that triggers the symptoms.

Is there a cure? For people like me this is the question that really matters. The answer on the day in February 1997 when I was immobilized by shakiness in the windowless room of the Washington bureau was an emphatic no. But some medications and procedures now in the pipeline at least give those of us with the disease an excuse for hoping that tomorrow's treatments will be ready for us when our illness is resistant to today's. Within eight months of the windowless room, the U.S. Food and Drug Administration had approved the first two new Parkinson's drugs in eight years. The two medications, which fool the brain into thinking they are a chemical that is in short supply in Parkinson's disease, promised little more than a modest improvement over two drugs that had been on the market for years. Still being tested, however, were much more futuristic treatments aimed at either repairing or re-placing the cells that have fallen victim to the disease. Researchers are trying to develop a reliable system for delivering chemicals called growth factors to the brain, where they hold out the prospect of restor-ing diseased brain cells to health. Another category of chemicals, the immunophilins, shows signs of doing the same. For replacement cells, researchers are exploring whether nerve cells from aborted fetuses can thrive when they are transplanted into diseased brains like mine. And with fetal tissue so politically sensitive because it comes from the prod-uct of abortions, stem cells—cells that can be coaxed into growing into almost any part of the body—are emerging as a possible source of nerve cells for transplantation. But stem cells have generated their own contro-versy because they mostly come from unwanted frozen embryos at fertility clinics. Finally, the discovery that faulty genes account for at least some cases of Parkinson's disease suggests that the ultimate cure for Parkinson's may come from gene therapy—the replacement of the bad genes with good ones.

The questions remain. But they were not on my mind after my first encounter with Dr. Reich. For the ensuing week, I was dazed. I couldn't eat. I couldn't sleep. I couldn't concentrate well enough to read. I couldn't face my office; I tried on the Wednesday and promptly turned around for home. I played a lot of solitaire in the early hours of the morning. Lots of people, I tried to convince myself, have Parkinson's disease—or worse—and manage to lead happy and productive lives. Why couldn't I? My thoughts on those long, dark February nights focused on how I was going to resume the routine of my life—or whether I could.

In My Doctors' Words
Dr. DC, May 19, 1989

Mr. Havemann is a 45-year-old man who presents with the chief complaint of a tremor. About nine months ago, he began to develop a tremor which has increased in intensity. The tremor primarily involves his right side, the leg more than the arm. He is right-handed. It does increase at times of stress. At times it is so severe that he is unable to write. . . . Recently he strained his back, but this is probably unrelated. . . .

On physical examination, Mr. Havemann was a pleasant, articulate man in no acute distress. His blood pressure was 125/80. His neck was supple. At rest and to varying degrees, he had a resting tremor which was quite coarse involving the entire right leg and foot. At times, the right hand would be involved, much less so was the left arm or leg involved.

IMPRESSION: Currently, Mr. Havemann has primarily a tremor that looks like an essential tremor. It is primarily unilateral but certainly is seen bilaterally. I think that this is more in the camp of an essential tremor. There is the family history, though the quality of his mother's tremor is different. . . . I have also put him on Inderal 60 mg [milligrams] per day as a diagnostic test for an essential tremor and have also asked him to try a strong drink of wine to see if this helps abate the tremor temporarily.

Biofeedback Specialist, December 20, 1989

This 46-year-old man reports a two-year history of tremor in his right arm, hand and leg. . . . Mr. Havemann also complains of muscle tension in his right arm and leg. Both the muscle tension and the tremor subsided as a result of the initial biofeedback session. Although he is somewhat skeptical about biofeedback, he has agreed to try it for six weeks and continue thereafter if it is helping.

Dr. DC, January 8, 1990

Inderal has helped his tremor but certainly has not abolished it. I am impressed today with the resting nature and coarseness of the tremor. In addition, there is some rigidity of the right arm. I am now actually thinking that this may be more of a parkinsonian-type tremor with a superimposed essential tremor. We do know that perhaps 10 percent of people with Parkinson's begin with an essential tremor.

Dr. Stephen G. Reich, February 5, 1990

Mr. Havemann's chief complaint is, "I can't stop shaking." . . . All fine motor tasks with the right hand (his dominant hand) are with greater effort. Writing is particularly problematic. . . . The tremor has been a major source of embarrassment, though, and he finds it distracting, has become self-conscious of it. He says that he would no longer go before a group to speak. He makes an effort to hide it by keeping his hands moving such as crossing them or actually sitting on his hands. His self-confidence has diminished because of the tremor. Emotionally, he is not depressed nor does he have any vegetative symptoms. . . .

Casual inspection reveals a thin man with an obvious tremor affecting the right upper and lower extremity. He looks very nervous. . . . Mental status, speech and language were normal as judged through casual conversation. Specifically, there was no voice tremor. . . .

The marked asymmetry of this tremor plus its occurrence primarily at rest in a pill-rolling morphology despite the increased frequency all point toward Parkinson's disease as its source, particularly coupled with diminished arm swing while walking. . . . In addition to the resting Parkinsonian tremor, though, there is a separate tremor of the upper extremities which is apparent with maintenance of a posture as well as with movement. Given his family history plus its longevity, this is an essential tremor. At this point, there are no symptoms or signs to suggest Parkinsonian syndrome other than idiopathic Parkinson's disease. . . .

Mr. Havemann is obviously disappointed as he was in hopes that I would have something different today, and specifically he fantasized that somehow or another his back spasms were connected to the tremor and that it would be an easy problem to cure. I educated him about the nature of Parkinson's disease as well as its very, very slow progression plus the fact that those patients who have predominantly tremor seem to fare better in the long run as compared to patients who have primarily akinesia [inability to move], rigidity and postural instability. I have also warned him that large amplitude tremors such as this are often very difficult to suppress. He has only been on the Artane [an anti-Parkinson's drug] for two weeks and, before making any medication changes, I would like to give it a bit longer to see its maximal effect. . . .

For the time being, though, the diagnosis has to sink in and it was obvious to me that Mr. Havemann is quite disturbed to hear about Parkinson's disease. His picture of his future has been clouded by mis-information and exposure to only some severe cases. I have empha-sized to him that the majority of patients actually lead a normal life span and do relatively well, albeit with medication. He has asked for some literature to read, and I have warned him to try not to focus on the worst possible outcomes. . . .

Mr. Havemann is still a little in doubt about the diagnosis and is concerned about follow-up care. . . . Should questions or problems come up before the appointment in a month, Mr. and Mrs. Havemann know how to reach me.

CHAPTER TWO

Myself before Parkinson's

Like any other major experience, illness actually changes us. . . . We enter
a realm of introspection and self-analysis. We think soberly, perhaps for
the first time, about our past and future. . . . Illness gives us that rarest
thing in the world— a second chance, not only at health but at life itself.
—Dr. Louis E. Bisch, "Turn Your Sickness into an Asset"

I'VE NEVER THOUGHT OF MYSELF AS especially introspective.
To me, introspection is psychological narcissism—a self-indulgence. A
favorite baseball player of mine, Jim Hickman, who played with the
Mets and the Cubs in the 1970s, was once asked what he was thinking as
thousands of fans cheered while he circled the bases after hitting a
game-winning home run during a tight pennant race. "Oh, nothing,"
Hickman replied. But at 3 o'clock in the morning, when you can't sleep
because you've just been told you have a degenerative disorder, it's hard
not to think about yourself. If nothing else, Parkinson's would force me
to learn a great deal about the kind of person I am. Some of it I would
like; some, I wouldn't. No matter. I couldn't escape myself.

Various people called or wrote during that first week to sympathize
or offer me encouragement, or both. I still have the cards. One call, from
an editor in Los Angeles, I remember particularly well not so much for
what he said as for how I replied. "It will be interesting to see how I deal
with this," I said, trying to achieve a journalistic detachment as an
observer rather than a participant. "I've never faced real adversity. My
parents are alive, and I've scarcely even been to a funeral. I wonder
what's going to happen now."

It was true: I had led an extraordinarily sheltered life. I grew up in the
1950s in the northern New Jersey bedroom suburbs of New York, where
the public school system was one of the hundreds that tell their students
they're the best schools in the country. (I know that because several of
my college classmates said they had been told the same thing.) I still
remember all but the opening line of my grade school song: "Dah de
dah de dah de dah, hurrah for Central School. We work and play the
livelong day, and obey the rules." The good kids didn't smoke—that
was against the rules—and the strongest mind-altering drink or drug

that anybody my age took was coffee. As an adolescent, I rebelled against my parents by going to church. On the day I was confirmed into the church, my mother actually showed up to watch, but my dad managed to be out of town on "business," thus maintaining his streak of several thousand Sundays without darkening a church door. In high school, my idea of challenging the conventional dress of the period—a sports shirt (with collar, of course) and wool or cotton trousers—was to wear a white shirt and tie.

All the while my mom and dad, in their own ways, protected me from the world around. Ruth was the kind of mother who has now virtually gone out of style. Extremely smart and well educated—she received a bachelor's degree from Washington University, in my family's home town of St. Louis, when she was 20—she married Dad, had me, and found herself home alone in our little suburb. She applied her intelligence and energy to the welfare of her only child. When I was found in grade school to be allergic to dust, she dusted and vacuumed my bedroom every day until I left for college. Until sometime during junior high school, she tucked me into bed every night. "Sleep tight," she would say, and when she got tired of saying that, she used words that rhymed ("Sleep right"; "Sleep light") until she ran out of rhymes, and then she shifted to "Sleep well" or "Sleep late." Even when I was an adult, she called me—when no one else was listening—her "boo-boo baby honey boy." I remember telling her once when I was a kid, "Mom, I hope I die before you, because I don't know what I'd ever do without you." She died when she was 79 and I was 49, and even though I was then living overseas and had a great job and a wonderful family of my own, for many weeks I felt lost without her.

My dad had his own ways of sheltering me from life's unpleasantness. To Dad, nothing was more unpleasant than old age and death. As far as I know, he didn't see his own father—a ne'er-do-well, overweight jockey whose only apparent influence on Dad was a love of horse racing—in the last ten years of his father's life. Dad was raised by his aunt in St. Louis after his parents divorced. I was in college when she died, and Dad actually went to St. Louis to put her affairs in order, but without taking Mom or me along. Mom and Dad also sheltered me from their own troubles. Both were in psychoanalysis for much of the time I was growing up—a fact that I learned only much later. Mom may or may not have had a drinking problem when I was an infant, first in New York and then in St. Louis, while Dad spent the last year of World War II writing press releases for the Army Air Force in Guam. But I do know this: All the while I was growing up, I never saw her take so much as a sip of beer. Dad, as it turned out, was a classic manic-depressive, but he hid it well. Before treatment with lithium became available, he would occasionally shut himself in the bedroom and cry until he had no tears left. But only once was I a witness, when he forgot to close the bedroom window while I was playing in the backyard.

Once in a rare while my parents would drive into New York City at night to go to dinner and see a Broadway show, usually a musical such as *Guys and Dolls* or *Damn Yankees*. As far back as I can remember, they never threw a party and never had anybody over for dinner—with the exception of relatives who had followed them from St. Louis to New York. Of these there were exactly three: my mother's older brother, Edgar Bohle, and his wife, Elinor, and Mom's younger brother, Bruce. They made a pretty remarkable group.

Dad was arguably the most successful magazine writer of his day, having moved to New York with *Time* magazine and then switched to *Life,* where he could make better use of his writing skills. Finally he left *Life* and became his own boss as a freelancer—and did so well that a *Time* profile in the 1960s dubbed him "King of the Lancers." His subjects ranged from Joe Welch, counsel for the U.S. Army and Sen. Joseph McCarthy's nemesis in the nationally televised Army-McCarthy hearings ("Senator, have you no shame?"), to Jayne Mansfield, the "dumb blonde" whom he revealed to be a closet intellectual. He traveled as far as Moscow, where both his stories and his photographs depicted the grimness of life in a totalitarian country. He was the first journalist given access to the 1948 Kinsey report on sexual behavior in the human male, in its time a shocking document for its matter-of-fact descriptions of premarital sex and homosexuality (subjects that today are on the cover of every magazine for teens). On rare occasions, Mom and I went along with Dad on his travels, as when he tried (unsuccessfully) to help former president Harry Truman write his memoirs when I was about 10. "Don't just mumble when you meet the president," Mom and Dad coached me. "Always answer him with, 'Yes, Mr. President' or 'No, Mr. President.'" They might as well have been talking to a stone. When Truman asked me if I liked Kansas City, or something like that, I mumbled, "Uh huh."

Writing was only half of Dad's life. He also was a dedicated horse-player and, starting in the mid-1950s, horse owner. In 1963 he reached the pinnacle of that world: one of his horses, a filly named Nubile, was among the best in the country and won about $60,000 in purses. Better yet, one afternoon he was the only bettor to pick as many as five of the winners of the last six races at Agua Caliente racetrack in Tijuana, Mexico. Not only did he collect $61,908.10, believed to have been the largest payoff on a $2 bet, but he also had the singular pleasure of writing an article about his feat in *Life*. With some justification, he proclaimed himself "the world's greatest handicapper."

Edgar, my mother's older brother, had helped raise his two younger siblings after their father died when Ed was a young teen. That experience helped turn Ed into an extremely serious and industrious adult. He worked in the public relations department of the chemical and drug manufacturer American Cyanamid, but he too had a passion for writing. While I was in high school and college, he published two mystery novels. His wife, Elinor, one of the rare professional women of her generation, was an extremely successful shoe designer. She spent much of her time in Italy while I was growing up. She and Ed wrote to each other virtually every day when she was overseas; when I cleaned out their apartment many years later, I came upon hundreds and hundreds of letters, all neatly saved and stored but never again to be read. They had no children, fearing that parenthood might interfere with Elinor's career. That seemed a pity; Ed seemed to relax and enjoy himself only when the family played multiple solitaire on our living room floor and, with a wide grin, he cried "Foul!" whenever anyone played a card before he could.

Bruce, my mother's younger brother, was so shy that he made me look like Dale Carnegie. A bachelor who was terrified of women, he moved to New York in 1953 to become editor of *Theatre Arts* magazine, a monthly published by the financier John D. MacArthur. Every month Theatre Arts published a new full-length play, a function that put Bruce in touch with Arthur Miller, Tennessee Williams, and Thornton Wilder. Bruce recounted some wonderful stories about MacArthur and his brother Charlie, who had teamed up with Ben Hecht to write *Front Page*, a classic play about the newspaper business in Chicago during Prohibition, and who later married the actress Helen Hayes. To Bruce, who was no flaming liberal himself, John D. MacArthur was a right-wing fanatic whose bull-headed independence was captured in his famous challenge, "If you're going to sue me, get in line."

In this tight-knit family, I felt special. I was an only child (and, I concluded much later, an unexpected one; why would my parents have had a child just when Dad might have to go off to World War II?). In fact, I was the only member of my generation in the entire family. My mother's two brothers were childless; so was her only cousin. On Dad's side, the closest thing I had to cousins my own age were the three children of his half-sister (Dad's mother having remarried after divorcing his father), but Dad scarcely communicated with anybody on his side of the family, and I saw my half-cousins no more than once or twice as a child. From my vantage point, I was the sole heir to the wisdom of my entire family. I believed that every candy bar I ate, every baseball I threw, and every comic book I read was privileged because it had been eaten, thrown, or read by me.

Privileged I was, but I was equally insulated. When I graduated from high school I had hardly ever had a date, much less a girlfriend. My rare attempts turned out disastrously: once I invited a girl to play tennis, but then, when a bunch of my friends turned up, I was so embarrassed to be seen with her that I played with the guys until she got tired of waiting and walked home. No more naïve 18-year-old ever arrived in Harvard Yard—except maybe my freshman roommate. We both must have asked the college housing office for the same kind of roommate: "Dweeb seeking even greater dweeb." Timothy Leary was just beginning to enlist students in his drug experiments, but at Harvard we were far from the cutting edge of the counterculture. When a roommate and I brought dates back to our room as juniors, we offered them a choice of Coke or 7-Up. I was Class of '65, meaning that I graduated just before the Vietnam War demonstrations. During my day, the target of student protests was the university's decision to switch its diplomas from Latin to English.

I managed to bluff my way through college as a math major, although it soon became clear that math was no way to earn a living. As the son of a journalist, I gravitated naturally to the student newspaper, the *Harvard Crimson*. Doubting that I could write well, I joined the paper's business staff. In my junior year no sports reporter wanted to cover the hockey team, and so I got my start as a journalist by writing about Gene Kinasewich and Ike Ikauniks and other luminaries of Harvard's strong team. Never once in two hockey seasons did I muster sufficient courage to actually talk to any of the players. Oddly enough, journalism attracts shy people—my father wasn't outgoing either—because it forces us to get out and talk to people. So after college I immediately became a reporter, starting my career at the Portland *Oregonian* for $100 a week ($2 more than a rank beginner's pay, the managing editor pointedly told me). My first assignment was to interview an amateur gardener who had grown an eighteen-petal lily—an extraordinary accomplishment, I was informed, considering that most lilies of that particular species had six petals and only a few had as many as twelve. For another assignment, an older reporter and I took the Scholastic Aptitude Tests. I don't remember what I wrote about the experience, but I do remember that I scored lower on the math test as a Harvard mathematics graduate than I had as a high school senior.

Portland was a lovely city to raise a family but a lousy one to find news, and after two years I landed a reporting job with the Chicago *Sun-Times*. No shortage of news there: within eighteen months I had covered the urban riots following the assassination of Dr. Martin Luther King and the police riots during the Democratic National Convention. Still I managed to glide through life without being personally bruised. I believe I once took a puff of a marijuana cigarette, but I had no idea how to inhale.

If ever adversity struck me, there was little chance that I would have a family of my own to comfort me. I was as shy as Einstein was smart. Women terrified me, just as girls had when I was a kid. I once spent an hour doggedly throwing a Frisbee back and forth with a young woman at a picnic that a mutual friend had set up, because I had no idea what else to do with her. I was tall, skinny, and awkward physically as well as socially. The likelihood that I would get to know someone well enough to marry her—and that she would want to have anything to do with me—seemed infinitely remote: about the same as the probability that the nine planets would arrange themselves in a precise straight line.

Early in 1969 the planets must have aligned. On one spring Monday, an editor ushered a new reporter to the desk behind mine, which had been vacant for two years. I was miffed because I had kept my copy paper on that desk. (In those days, we actually wrote on paper.) When my new neighbor, whose byline was Judy Nicol, offered to let me keep the paper on her desk, I figured she had to be all right. Besides, she was married and had a young daughter; that made her less threatening. So I got to know her reasonably well—well enough that as her marriage fell apart, I felt more comfortable with her than I ever had with any single woman of my age. Still more extraordinary, she seemed interested in me. Luckily, she valued intellect over appearance. So I courted her by showing her how to prove that the square root of two is an irrational number (that is, it can't be written as a fraction) and discussing recent discoveries about DNA. When she and her daughter, Theresa, moved from their house in the suburbs to a one-bedroom apartment just north of downtown Chicago, her moving crew consisted of me and the features editor. The features editor left, but I didn't. It took us a couple of years, but we finally married in my parents' house on the day after the 1972 Watergate burglary, an event that didn't register on our radar screen. More important was the weekend's other big story, Hurricane Agnes, which closed the New York airports on the day we were supposed to begin our honeymoon and, when we got a flight the next day, followed us all the way to Quebec City, undoubtedly the first hurricane since the Ice Age ever to go so far north. (It forced us to spend much of the first few days of our honeymoon in our cozy hotel room—there are worse fates.) Soon after we returned to Chicago, I was offered a job in Washington reporting for a magazine, then totally obscure and now somewhat less so, called *National Journal.* Judy quickly landed a reporting job at the *Washington Post.* The three of us were installed in a rented suburban split-level in time for Theresa to begin the fifth grade in 1973.

As was then true for many teens, Theresa had a rocky adolescence. But she pulled herself together in her last two years of high school and won admission to the University of California, Berkeley. In her second year, she decided (with no prodding from us) to be a doctor. Within another decade, completing one of the greatest comebacks since Bobby Thomson's ninth-inning home run beat the Brooklyn Dodgers in 1951, she graduated from the George Washington University medical school.

Theresa's adolescence had discouraged Judy and me from having more children. Her turnaround changed our minds. Anne was born in 1981 and Margaret and William followed four years later. In between, I switched to the Washington bureau of the *Los Angeles Times.* In our only brush with child-related adversity, Will was born without the usual soft spot on top of his head. Without surgery, his head would grow in the front and back but not on the sides; he would have an elongated skull that, while probably doing no harm to his brain, would leave him looking mildly freakish. Much as our pediatric neurosurgeon assured us that the operation would be routine, shaving away the bone on top of an infant's head seemed terrifying to us. The operation lasted about an hour. Afterward we found Will lying on a rolling hospital bed, his skin as white as the sheet beneath him. When the doctor slammed his hand down on the bed as hard as he could, Will barely budged. The doctor took that to be a good sign. We didn't. Would he survive the night? (Would we?) He did. The next day his big brown eyes were as wide as they had been before the operation. Since then, the kids' most serious health problems haven't been much more than an ear infection.

This all made for a pleasant life. But it did not prepare me for the verdict from Dr. Reich that February morning in 1990. As I brooded in the nights that followed, I wondered how I could resume the routine of my life—or whether I could. Lots of people, I told myself as I lost one solitaire game after another, have Parkinson's disease—or worse—and still lead happy and productive lives. In a muddled way, I tried to sort out the available strategies. Religion wasn't available to me. Despite having gone to church in my adolescent rebellion, I ultimately adopted my parents' antipathy toward organized religion.

Still, you don't have to be religious to believe that life has some transcendent purpose, that we are all here for a reason. My personal philosophy is best expressed by the contemporary British zoologist Richard Dawkins, who argues that people (and all other living things) are machines to ensure the survival and reproduction of their genes. The most successful genes, Dawkins writes, are those that encase themselves in bodies that are most likely to survive and reproduce. "The first survival machines probably consisted of nothing more than a protective coat," he writes. "But making a living got steadily harder as new rivals arose with better and more effective survival machines. Survival machines got bigger and more elaborate, and the process was cumulative and progressive."[1] Evolution is what he's talking about, and to me it provides a compelling explanation of how we got where we are.

If Dawkins is right, it follows (at least to me) that a sensible life's goal is to care as best as I can for those who share some of my genes— namely, my children. As long as they need me, I want to be there for them. I want to provide them with the psychological and financial support they'll need to become good citizens of the United States and the world. I ultimately discovered that I couldn't properly tend to my children's needs without understanding my own. Doing that required learning more about the part of me where something had gone so terribly wrong—the brain.

CHAPTER THREE

The Magnificent Brain

If the human brain were so simple that we could understand it,
we would be so simple that we couldn't.
—Emerson M. Pugh, engineer

ON NOVEMBER 22, 1963, the day President John F. Kennedy
was assassinated, I was a junior at Harvard, his alma mater. The news
stopped campus life cold. Students mourned, they grieved, they got
drunk. I went immediately to the offices of the *Crimson,* the student
newspaper. Some of us generally devoted more time to the *Crimson*
than to classes, and we knew immediately what to do: put out an extra
edition. Instead of mourning or grieving or drinking, we called prominent people for their reaction and researched Kennedy's life. We wrote
stories, composed headlines, selected pictures, and attended to all the
mechanical details of publishing a newspaper. In short, we escaped
from reality by plunging headlong into it. So it has been with me and
Parkinson's.

I have finally forced myself to learn the basics of the disease only by
treating it as an urgent story that needs reporting.[1] Nine years after Dr.
Reich's diagnosis, as I write this, I have engaged the disease as an
investigator, detective, and observer—not as a patient seeking information about his own condition. This has given me license to explore
things that would otherwise be difficult. Delving into Parkinson's has
turned out to be like diving into the New Jersey surf in the spring:
breathtakingly cold at first but, after the initial shock, bracing and rewarding. When I controlled my personal dread of Parkinson's, I found
that the disease was causing me to ask new questions and examine new
subjects. The process, both exciting and sobering, leads inevitably to
the brain.

We take the brain for granted. It's a scant three pounds of cells
floating in four or five ounces of a briny fluid inside the skull. But just
about everything we do, think, and feel depends on the brain's working
well. It collects our thoughts and our emotions. It regulates how fast our
heart beats and how much sugar gets to our muscles. It remembers how
to solve quadratic equations (if we're lucky) and what we were doing the

day Kennedy was shot (if we're old enough). It controls our fingers when we thread a needle and our arms and legs when we do a somersault. All this we regard as routine, as everyone's birthright—and that's just as well. If we thought about it at all, we'd be amazed that nature had developed anything so intricate and complex, yet so efficient and compact. Having learned what I have learned, I'm just glad that most of my brain works most of the time.

The popular comparison of the brain to a computer insults the brain. True, some superficial similarities exist. Both accept information from the outside world—"input." Both process this information by converting it into electrical impulses that travel along particular pathways. Both make decisions—"output"—according to the results of this information processing. But the differences dwarf the similarities. The computer is bullheaded. If your name is Smith but you type in Snith, it won't know who you are. The brain has no trouble spotting the typo and fixing it. The computer is pedestrian. It can easily memorize a twenty-digit number but can't figure out the moral of Little Red Riding Hood. The brain understands what the Wolf is up to even if it can't keep all the digits straight in a twenty-digit number. The computer functions according to how it was programmed. By contrast, the brain can change its program—and constantly does.

The brain amazes not only by what it does but by how. In the computer, the electrical impulses take the form of electrons traveling at nearly the speed of light. The pathways are microscopic electrical circuits etched onto silicon chips. Along the pathways are a host of branches in the road, controlled by switches. Whether the electrical impulse takes the left fork or the right fork depends on whether the switch is on or off.

In the brain, the process is far more complex. The brain's circuits are formed by living cells called nerve cells, or neurons. The typical human brain contains something like fifty billion of them. (By comparison, there are about six billion people alive in the world today.) And each nerve cell is fabulously more complicated than a computer's digital switch. Within each tiny cell, messages are transmitted not by electrons but by electrically charged versions of several common elements— sodium, potassium, calcium, and chlorine. These charged particles are called ions. They do not actually travel up and down the nerve cell, the way electrons travel up and down a wire. Rather, they move back and forth between the nerve cell and the fluid that fills the space between the cells. Have you ever been to a sporting event where the crowd stands up and sits down in a pattern that makes a human wave? Nobody actually moves to the left or the right, but from a distance it looks as if a wave of standing people is moving around the stadium. The same effect can be achieved with a row of lights: if they turn on and off in the right pattern, the lights seem to move up or down the row. That's how nerve cells work. The ions of sodium and potassium and calcium and chlorine do not move up and down the nerve cell; they move in and out of the nerve cell through the cell membrane. But the pattern is equivalent to the movement of an electrical charge along the length of the nerve cell right up to its end.

Or, to be precise, its many ends. The average nerve cell in the brain has something like 10,000 ends! Half of them are receptors, receiving information from other, nearby nerve cells, and the other half are transmitters, sending messages. (See figure 3.1.) Each receptor is capable of receiving one or the other of two basic messages: one message tending to turn the nerve cell on and one tending to turn it off. About 1,000 times a second, the cell weighs the totality of "on" and "off" messages. If the "offs" outnumber the "ons," the nerve cell does nothing. But if the "ons" dominate, the nerve cell fires off a message to its transmitter ends. When you consider that the brain has some 50 billion nerve cells, that each one is connected to something like 10,000 others, and that each one can fire some 1,000 times a second, you begin to appreciate the brain's extraordinary power. I feel I've lost my excuse for not remembering my wedding anniversary (but Judy can't remember it either) or the capital of Tennessee (Nashville, not Knoxville).

Actually, the nerve cells are not exactly connected to one another. There is a tiny gap between the transmitter end of one nerve cell and the receiver end of another. This gap—about twenty one-millionths of a millimeter from one side to the other—is known as a synapse. When the "wave" of ions reaches the transmitter end of one nerve cell, it does not jump the gap. Rather, it causes the release of a chemical stored in a little sac. The chemical, like a swimmer taking the baton in a relay race, carries the message across the synapse to the receiving end of the next nerve cell.

What happens next depends on the shapes of the chemical relay-swimmer and the waiting receptor. If the relay-swimmer doesn't fit into the receptor, nothing happens at all. But if it does, it touches off an electrical wave along this next nerve cell. And the cycle begins all over again. Eventually the message reaches its ultimate destination: perhaps the leg, where the message might be to run like crazy; or perhaps the

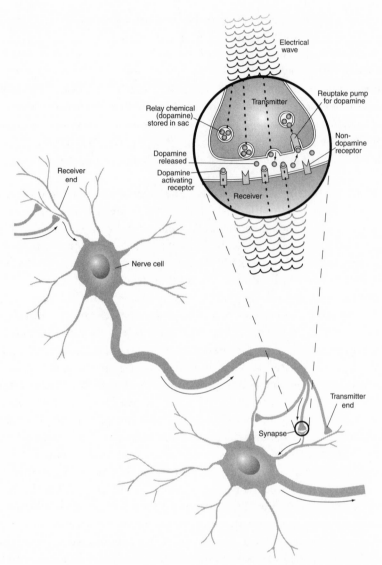

Figure 3.1. Each nerve cell, or neuron, in the brain has thousands of processes that collect information from "upstream" nerve cells and thousands more that transmit information to "downstream" nerve cells. The nerve cells are separated by tiny gaps, called synapses. Chemical messengers called neurotransmitters carry messages across the synapses from one nerve cell to the next. The neurotransmitters are manufactured in the nerve cells and stored there, in tiny sacs, until they are needed. After each use, many of the neurotransmitter molecules are pumped back into the transmitter nerve cell and start the cycle over again. Dopamine is one such neurotransmitter.

brain itself, where the message might be to remember to buy a gallon of milk on the way home from work.

None of these messages would get through without the chemicals that serve as the relay-swimmers across the synapses. Without them, the brain could not function; nerve cells would have no way of transmitting their message to the next nerve cells down the line. Altogether, scientists have identified about ten kinds of these chemicals, although many more are believed to exist. One disease in particular is known to result from a shortage of one of them. That disease is Parkinson's, and the chemical is dopamine.

Dopamine is manufactured in several parts of the brain. But for the Parkinson's story, the place that matters the most is the substantia nigra—Latin for "black substance," so called because of its heavy concentration of black pigment. The substantia nigra (which actually comes in two parts, one on each side of the brain) is a long, skinny mass of nerve cells about the shape of a bread stick, although much smaller and tapered at the ends. It is strategically located deep in the brain underneath the huge lobes of gray and white matter that are responsible for humans' unique ability to think. (See figure 3.2.) This part of the brain is called the midbrain, and the circuits passing through it (many of which bypass the substantia nigra) mostly control muscle movement. When we consciously order our legs to run, the message flows from the cerebral cortex (the thinking part of the brain) through the substantia nigra and back to the cortex before finally traveling to the legs. Likewise, the substantia nigra plays a critical role in subconscious movement—for example, when we walk without thinking about it. The circuitry in this part of the brain is extraordinary in its complexity. Figure 3.3A is a simplified (!) wiring diagram, while figure 3.3B shows how Parkinson's disrupts the brain's circuitry, culminating in excessive inhibition of activity in the thalamus.

The nerve cells in the substantia nigra manufacture their own dopamine from an amino acid called tyrosine. We get the tyrosine from the protein we eat. A typical hamburger, for example, contains one to two grams of tyrosine. Turning tyrosine into dopamine is a two-step process. First tyrosine becomes a compound that is usually called levodopa and sometimes called L-dopa. Then levodopa is converted into dopamine. Each step takes place only in the presence of a special kind of protein called an enzyme. (To see all this in schematic form, examine figure 3.4.)

Dopamine is scarce even in a healthy brain. If you could isolate the

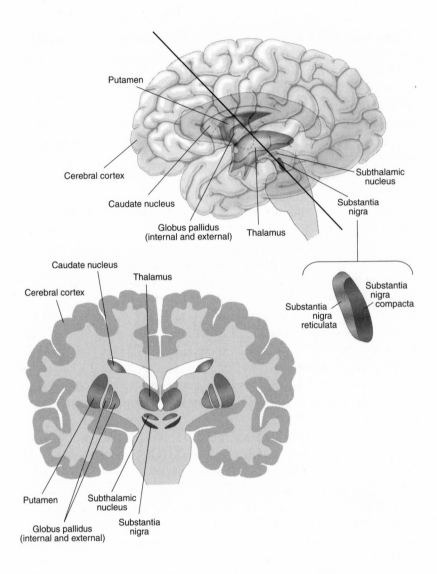

Figure 3.2. A side view of the brain shows that all the major brain structures involved in Parkinson's disease are located deep inside. The bold diagonal line in the top illustration shows the plane of the bottom illustration. The substantia nigra is the most important structure in Parkinson's disease. There is a substantia nigra on each side of the brain, and each one comes in two parts, the compacta and the reticulata. The pattern of cell death in the substantia nigra influences the symptoms of each individual with Parkinson's.

brain's many constituent chemicals, about five parts of every million would be dopamine: because the brain weighs about one and a third kilograms (the metric equivalent of three pounds), that means about seven milligrams of dopamine. How much is that? Well, some years ago Judy and I were vacationing in Turkey, and Judy decided to buy some cumin at an open-air spice market. Like most countries except the United States, Turkey uses the metric system. Judy, however, is a die-hard devotee of the American way. So when the spice-shop proprietor asked how much she wanted, she knew only that she didn't want much—and she held up a single finger. So the poor young fellow measured out exactly one gram of cumin, which was hardly anything. Seven milligrams, then, is seven one-thousandths of hardly anything. Even if it could all be collected in one place, you'd have a hard time seeing it with an unaided eye.

No wonder dopamine is scarce. In its precarious environment, individual molecules survive, on average, no more than a few seconds, or about the time it will take you to read this sentence. After they are manufactured inside a substantia nigra cell, molecules of dopamine are stored like clusters of grapes in the tiny sacs found at each of the cell's many transmitting ends. Chances are that within a second, an electrical message will come flashing along the nerve cell, and the sacs will dump their contents into the tiny synapse. Most of the dopamine molecules will swim to a receptor waiting on the other side. Scientists have identified five distinct receptors that provide a snug fit for dopamine molecules. Two of these receptors interpret the dopamine as an "on" messenger; they signal their nerve cell to send messages to the next nerve cells in the network. The other three respond to the dopamine with the opposite result: they send a signal encouraging their nerve cell to remain inactive. In either case, however, the dopamine molecules hook onto the receptors for only a brief moment before the receptors, in a flash, hurl them back into the fluid that bathes the brain. Most of the dopamine molecules are pumped back into the cell where they were manufactured, and the cycle starts all over. But sometimes they are picked off by one of two enzymes that lurk in this part of the brain.[2] (See figure 3.5.) The enzymes transform dopamine into a useless chemical that is ultimately flushed out of the body. On any given trip, the chances are about four out of five that a dopamine molecule will evade its predators and make it back to its home nerve cell safely. But that means each dopamine molecule has scarcely more than a 50-50 chance of surviving three plunges into the synapse. Only about one molecule in ten is likely

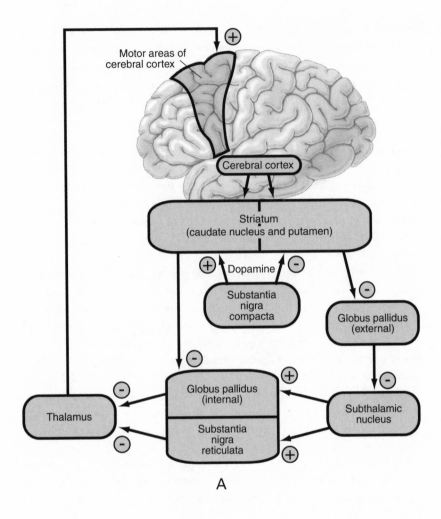

Figure 3.3. *A,* When a command (such as "run") originates in the cerebral cortex (the thinking part of the brain), it triggers a cascade of electrical signals, some of which pass through the substantia nigra before looping back to the motor area of the cortex and finally traveling to the body—in this case, the legs. *B,* Lacking in dopamine, the substantia nigra compacta in Parkinson's disease fails to transmit its messages, some stimulatory and some inhibitory, to the striatum. This sets off several sequences of garbled messages, culminating in too much inhibition of the thalamus and, consequently, too little activation of the cerebral cortex.

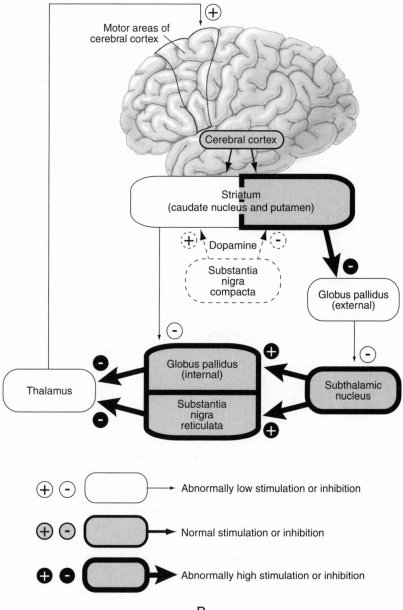

Motor areas of
cerebral cortex

Cerebral cortex

Striatum
(caudate nucleus and putamen)

Dopamine

Substantia
nigra
compacta

Globus pallidus
(external)

Globus pallidus
(internal)

Substantia
nigra
reticulata

Thalamus

Subthalamic
nucleus

⊕ ⊖ ⟶ Abnormally low stimulation or inhibition

⊕ ⊖ ⟶ Normal stimulation or inhibition

⊕ ⊖ ⟶ Abnormally high stimulation or inhibition

B

Figure 3.4. Tyrosine, a common amino acid, is converted in the substantia nigra first to levodopa (L-dopa) and then to dopamine. At each stage, an enzyme acts as a catalyst: it facilitates the transformation without losing its own identity. Tyrosine hydroxylase is the enzyme that converts tyrosine to levodopa. L-AAAD is the enzyme that turns levodopa into dopamine.

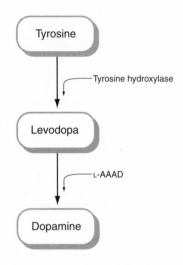

to survive ten trips. Since each round trip takes about a second, that means that nine molecules out of ten are eliminated within ten seconds.[3]

At its prime, the substantia nigra contains only about 450,000 dopamine-producing nerve cells. That is something less than 0.001 percent of all the brain's nerve cells. Even in the healthiest persons, the nerve cells that produce dopamine slowly die. In most people, the cells die too slowly to make a difference. In some, they die much more quickly. Those that remain do their best to compensate for their shrinking numbers by boosting production as much as fivefold. But when only about 20 percent of the cells are left, they cannot manufacture enough dopamine to swim all the relays that dopamine should. (See figure 3.6.) The result: many of the brain's messages to the muscles can't get through, and there is a general disruption of the ability to move normally. Most commonly, the arms and legs tremble while resting but not while moving. Many muscles and joints grow stiff. Movement is difficult and slow. Posture deteriorates. People with these symptoms have Parkinson's disease.

Why are my dopamine-producing nerve cells dying faster than, say, Judy's? Neurological journals are littered with studies that contradict each other. People who live on farms and handle pesticides and herbicides are more likely to get Parkinson's than those who live in cities—or people who live in cities are just as likely to get the disease as those who live on farms. Head injuries put people at risk for Parkinson's—or there is no correlation between head injuries and Parkinson's. Exposure to industrial toxins is a risk factor for Parkinson's—or industrial toxins are

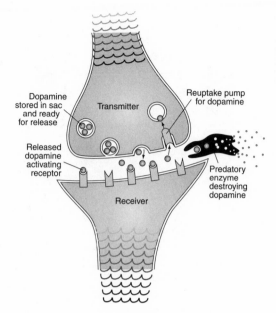

Dopamine stored in sac and ready for release

Transmitter

Reuptake pump for dopamine

Released dopamine activating receptor

Predatory enzyme destroying dopamine

Receiver

Figure 3.5. In the synapses, predatory enzymes called COMT and MAO-B convert levodopa into useless chemicals.

not associated with Parkinson's. There are even some generally unhealthy activities—smoking and drinking coffee—that, according to some studies but not others, protect against Parkinson's. Or could it be the other way around: could people with a dopamine deficit be inclined not to like tobacco and coffee?[4]

As a result of the confusion, many of us with Parkinson's have our own individual hunches about what brought on the disease. It's a special puzzle because we may have contacted the poison—assuming there is one—years and years before developing symptoms. Larry McCurdy, a member of my Parkinson's support group, remembers that his finger used to twitch after he used it to press the nozzle on cans of spray paint, as he often did as a young man. Could the chemicals in the spray have brought on the Parkinson's that he developed in his 50s? Mike, a member of a different support group, grew up in Utah during World War II, and his prime suspect is radiation drifting over his home from nuclear weapons tests in neighboring Nevada. My imagined villains are the little balls of mercury that I touched in high school chemistry class. Could that liquid metal, known now (but not then) to be toxic in so many other ways, have begun the assault on my brain?[5] Only recently have scientists begun to understand the mechanism by which the brain cells die.[6]

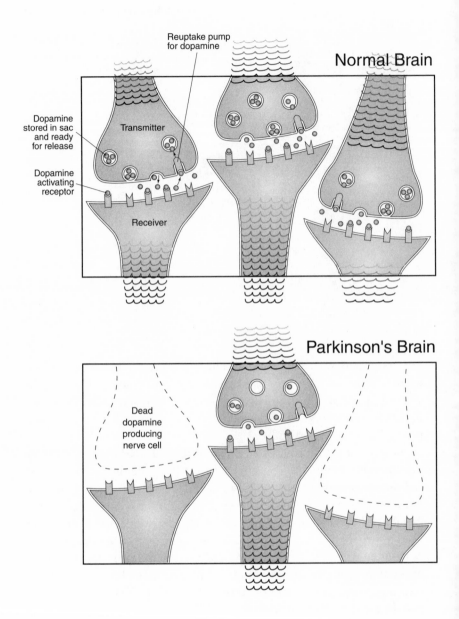

Figure 3.6. In Parkinson's disease, many of the substantia nigra nerve cells are dead or dying and produce little dopamine to influence downstream nerve cells.

Indeed, in about 20 percent of cases diagnosed as Parkinson's disease, the patients turn out not to have Parkinson's at all but rather another, usually more severe neurological disorder. It is generally clear within a couple of years whether what had been thought to be Parkinson's is really "Parkinson's plus." So there are plenty of explanations for Dr. DC's difficulty diagnosing my condition. A recent European survey found that one-quarter of all Parkinson's cases had gone undetected until researchers went house to house looking for them.[7] The only sure sign of Parkinson's is the presence of mysterious little knots of pinkish protein (called Lewy bodies) in dying substantia nigra cells. Unfortunately, these can be found only in an autopsy.

Parkinson's symptoms can vary widely from one individual to the next, perhaps reflecting different patterns of cell death in the substantia nigra and other dopamine-producing areas of the brain. In my case, the tremor was the most obvious early symptom, although the muscles of my arms and legs grew stiff and rigid and my posture deteriorated. Slowness of movement, the last of the four cardinal signs of Parkinson's, became significant only several years after my diagnosis. The tremor is Parkinson's signature symptom, although not everyone with Parkinson's develops one. It's hard to miss: when I rest my hands on my legs while I'm sitting, they tremble in a way that looks as if I'm rolling pills between my fingers. It goes away when I move and when I sleep—and I have to be extremely tired before my legs stop shaking and allow me to sleep. Although the tremor's precise mechanism remains obscure, this much is clear: it develops when muscles receive an abnormal signal from the brain because there is not enough dopamine to relay the normal signal. Most muscles that move body parts come in pairs, one to extend whatever the muscle is attached to and one to bend (flex) it. In the arm, for example, the triceps extends the forearm and the biceps bends it. In healthy people, the brain, which is in constant communication with these pairs of muscles, ordinarily keeps each muscle slightly engaged—the reason their elbows and knees and knuckles are slightly bent when at rest. In Parkinson's patients, the two muscles governing each limb instead contract alternately: first one, then the other. Why the muscles behave this way—why, for example, they don't contract at the same time or simply go limp—is not known. What is known is that the alternate contractions of opposing muscles such as the biceps and the triceps result in the familiar Parkinson's tremor.

Classic Parkinson's usually develops according to one of two patterns, although there is considerable overlap. In one, the predominant problems are with posture, balance, and gait. The second is dominated by the tremor. Those like me for whom the tremor is paramount typically develop Parkinson's at a younger age than those whose greater challenges are sitting, standing, and walking normally. On the other hand, our form of the disease tends to progress more slowly and impair our ability to get along less severely, and it is less likely to lead to dementia.

I count myself lucky that my brand of Parkinson's disease is the least destructive kind. And I regard myself as luckier still that insufficient dopamine production in the substantia nigra affects mostly movement rather than mental faculties. The symptoms of many other chemical imbalances in the brain are mental. Alzheimer's disease, manic-depressive disorder, and schizophrenia are now known to have chemical origins; in fact, an excess of dopamine in another part of the brain altogether is thought to play a role in some forms of schizophrenia.

In the end, I suspect, everything the brain does will turn out to have a chemical basis. It does not seem necessary to invoke some kind of supernatural explanation; the brain's chemicals routinely perform miraculous feats. To believe otherwise, in my view, is to believe that there can be effects with no natural causes: the equivalent of believing that you can read other people's minds by concentrating hard enough on their brain waves; that the alignment of the planets influences your sexual prowess; that water can suddenly be made into wine. All these would be spectacular if true. But I find the world we can see and hear and smell and touch to be far more interesting than imagined mysteries. This is what science is about. The ordinary world around us may not be stranger than fiction, but it is more wonderful—in the original, literal sense of that word.

Does this make us the pawns of our brain's chemistry, acting out a script dictated by our own particular collection of mental molecules? When we do wrong, can we protest, "My dopamine made me do it"? Not at all. To say that chemicals are the agents of the brain's commands is not to say that chemicals are the initiators of those commands. Our values and morals are no more determined by our mental chemistry than they are imprinted on our genes. Free will still has a place: it is what, in the first instance, sets these chemicals in motion. Granted, our own particular chemical makeup limits the behaviors available to us. No matter how hard he tried and how many psychoanalysts he saw, my father could not shake his depressions simply by willing them away. I might even be convinced that a chemical disorder in the brain compelled John Hinckley to shoot President Ronald Reagan. I am certain, however, that people whose brain chemicals are within a normal range have the capacity to decide whether to follow behind Mother Teresa or Jack the Ripper.

Nor does the brain's chemical basis strip it of its majesty, of its capacity to inspire wonder. Quite the contrary. Parkinson's disease has led me, however unwittingly, to regard the brain with the same sort of awe that I once reserved for the vastness of the universe. What seems astonishing is that a mere three-pound object, made of the same atoms that constitute everything else under the sun, is capable of directing virtually everything that humans have done: flying to the moon and hitting seventy home runs, writing *Hamlet* and building the Taj Mahal —even unlocking the secrets of the brain itself.

In My Doctors' Words
Dr. Stephen G. Reich, February 27, 1990

Since I saw Mr. Havemann originally, he has had a chance to do quite a bit of reading about Parkinson's disease and seems to have acclimated fairly well to the idea of having it. He mentions that he does get nervous when thinking about his future or his overall condition. . . . He was very honest with his co-workers in explaining his diagnosis and, as such, does not face the burden of having to hide it from others. He says that additionally, he is not making much of a conscious effort to hide his tremor. . . . Even the embarrassment which had been a problem previously has improved somewhat. He asked a number of questions today based on his reading, and we spent a long time discussing the pathogenesis and treatment of Parkinson's disease. He remains completely functional with regard to his activities of daily living and, overall, feels relatively happy with the current state of things. He says that if he could remain at his current state for the next 30 to 40 years, he would be content. He does have a bit more trouble shaving, cuts himself more often than he used to. Writing is still a problem, and it is more difficult to brush his teeth. . . . He is holding up relatively well emotionally with no symptoms or signs to suggest depression.

CHAPTER FOUR

Escaping Abroad

> Those who visit foreign nations, but associate only with their own
> countrymen, change their climate, but not their customs. They see new
> meridians but the same men; and with heads as empty as their pockets,
> return home with traveled bodies, but nontraveled minds.
> —Charles Caleb Colton, English clergyman

APPRECIATING THE BRAIN was not high on my to-do list immediately after Dr. Reich's unwelcome news on February 5, 1990. First I
had to decide what to do with my life. In the week that followed, I
subconsciously adopted a strategy of living as if I had no disease at all.
Later I would join a support group for people who contracted Parkinson's disease at a young age, and I would learn much from it. But then,
in early 1990, I wanted nothing to do with other people with Parkinson's. They only reminded me of my condition. The only support
groups I wanted were my family, my friends, and my job. Just by being
there, Judy and the children reminded me that I still had a lot to live for.
I couldn't pretend that I was still healthy if worrying wouldn't let me get
a night's sleep. Judy and the children treated me normally, and that—as
much as anything else—nudged me back to normalcy.

Friends helped too. When I failed to show up at work for an entire
week after my Monday morning diagnosis, two reporters visited the
house on the weekend—one on Saturday, one on Sunday—and stayed
for several hours to make sure I didn't become a hermit. That meant a
lot. As it happened, Judy and I had been invited to a third reporter's
house for dinner that Saturday. I didn't feel up to it, but Judy said I
couldn't hide forever. She was right. It turned out to be like any other
dinner party—which made it hugely memorable. I didn't spill food on
my lap. I didn't shake my drink out of its glass. Everyone there knew
about my Parkinson's. No one talked about it. That was how I wanted
it. Fortified, I made it to work the following Monday. Everything went
fine.

Actually, better than fine. Only later did I learn that many employers
do not give Parkinson's patients much opportunity. The disease scares
them too: it conjures up visions of disabled workers disrupting everyday

business by not carrying their share of the work. The *Los Angeles Times* had no such misgivings—or, if it did, I never learned of them. Just the opposite, it seemed. A few weeks later, the paper decided to station an economics reporter in Brussels, the headquarters of the European Union (then called the European Community). At the time, the twelve nations of the European Community were completing their creation of a single economic market, without tariffs or other national trade barriers. Surely this was my last chance to be a foreign correspondent, a longtime ambition. The job played to my strengths. As a reporter and editor, I had specialized in economics. I even knew some French—one of Belgium's two official languages (the other being Dutch)—from high school. The *Times* encouraged me to apply.

I knew without having to ask that Judy would be eager to try something new. After seventeen years of marriage, having brought Theresa through adolescence and given birth to three children of our own, we understood each other in ways that didn't require words. One thing I had learned about her was that she liked to try new things. Having grown up in a family that served potatoes three meals a day, she liked new dishes and new flavors. My illness compounded this impulse. She knew that my infirmities would limit her future just as surely as mine. Brussels was not only my last chance to live overseas. It was also hers, and she didn't have to tell me that she would leap at the prospect.

Judy had switched from editing to reporting at the *Washington Post* when William and Margaret were born, because an editor's hours consumed too much time. The *Post* had assigned her to a new beat on how the federal government manages itself. (Her conclusion: poorly.) She had done sensationally, thoroughly exploring and intimidating the obscure agencies that manage the government, producing stories where none had seemed to exist. She had a particularly good run of stories about the General Services Administration, which oversees the government's thousands of office buildings. As it happened, she completed several stories without personally meeting the top GSA managers. But the stories had been so pointed and incisive that, when she finally interviewed the head of the GSA, he and his staff were expecting a descendant of the Amazons. Imagine their chagrin when in walked a soft-spoken and pleasant woman who, without high heels, measured 4 feet 11 inches.

After four years of the bureaucracy beat, however, Judy had tired of it—so much so that, for the first time since her sophomore year in college, she was willing to relinquish a regular paycheck. She was entitled to feel weary. For all her life she had pedaled uphill. Judy grew up on a farm in northern Michigan that her grandfather had acquired for free in a land grant signed by President Rutherford B. Hayes. As farmland, the acreage was worth what it cost. It hardly mattered that the soil was too sandy to support most crops; the growing season that far north was too short to grow much of anything even in good soil. Judy's half-Scottish and half-German father, the eighth of her grandparents' nine children, worked the fields as hard and as well as was humanly possible. In good years, he broke even. Her mother, a graduate of Oberlin College in Ohio (she graduated in 1929, just in time for the Depression), was probably the best-educated person in the county. She brought in a regular income by teaching school.

Judy disliked almost everything about rural Michigan. She hated the poverty that trapped families in rickety trailers. She railed at the schools for being so narrow-minded as to punish her brother for allowing his hair to touch his ears. She even got tired of her name. Thanks to Judy Garland, *Judy* enjoyed a blaze of popularity in the 1940s; in an elementary class of eight or ten students, she was one of two Judys. Like a prisoner who obsessively files through the cell bars, Judy spent her high school years preparing to escape. She won every academic award in her high school and, by virtue of her cooking and sewing skills, was a 4-H champion of Michigan. (She still makes spectacular piecrust.) All that, plus good scores on the National Merit Scholarship test, earned her a full scholarship to Michigan State. There she dated someone in her Russian class and, before she had finished her first year of college, she had married him and had a baby. In fact, she took a midterm exam within days of giving birth. For the rest of her college years, while I enjoyed the carefree life at Harvard with parents paying the freight, Judy raised her daughter and eventually worked as a reporter at the Jackson *Citizen Patriot*—even as she maintained a full academic schedule and earned an A average.

Nor were our children an obstacle to moving. In many ways, they are so different from their parents—and each other—that they scarcely seem like siblings. Anne is a particularly strong reader and writer, but highly disorganized. Margaret is practical, handy, and managerial. Will, easygoing and personable but occasionally careless, enjoys acting and singing in front of audiences. At their ages in 1990—Anne was 8 and the twins were 4—they could be uprooted without a steam shovel or an act of Congress. William and Margaret were just completing nursery

school, and Anne was in the second grade at the Washington Interna-
tional School, a private school that offered bilingual programs in French
and Spanish. (We had cleverly chosen Spanish on the theory that it
would be more useful.) So I applied for the Brussels job. Just when
most workers with Parkinson's have to fight demotion or dismissal, I
was vying for a plum assignment.

My bosses in Los Angeles didn't ignore my health; they wondered if
somebody with Parkinson's disease could manage three arduous years
as a foreign correspondent. I wasn't certain myself, but Dr. Reich encouraged me. He said the odds were good that I'd be only marginally
shakier after three years than I was then—which wasn't much, except
when under high stress. Unfortunately, nothing was so stressful as having to discuss the cloud over my future. During a crucial meeting with
Shelby Coffey, the newspaper's top editor, I shook so hard that I almost
exploded out of my chair. Nevertheless, Shelby heard me out, and I
became one of two finalists. The foreign editor wanted the other candidate. But Shelby overruled him, despite the shaky interview. "If it didn't
work," he told me later, "we could always regroup. As it turned out, I
never had reason to regret it."

The foreign editor, my new boss, never even hinted that my selection
disappointed him. He allowed our family about three months to prepare
for the assignment, and I started four hours of daily language lessons
from a French embassy official's wife. If she aimed to humiliate me, she
succeeded magnificently. After several weeks, she read me a simple
paragraph in French and asked me several questions. I couldn't understand them, much less answer. "C'est une catastrophe," she said over
and over. That was one French word I understood the first time.

In Brussels on a house-hunting trip, my tremor was moderate but
sufficiently noticeable that our real estate agent, whose brother had
Parkinson's, immediately guessed my condition. She located just the
house Judy and I wanted: a turn-of-the-century *art nouveau* townhouse
in a neighborhood where few expatriate Americans lived. The house
(which had probably been built with the wealth looted from the Belgian
Congo) was narrow, deep, and extremely tall. The ceilings were high
enough to accommodate two professional basketball players, one standing on the other's shoulders. Anne, the mistress of the top floor,
counted seventy-four stairs from the front door to her bed. Recently the
building had been divided into four tenements, but a wealthy Finnish
television broadcaster had bought it and, having gutted everything but

the facade and the load-bearing walls, completely rebuilt the inside. For the next three years we would live here, on the Rue du Mont-Blanc in the neighborhood of St. Gilles.

Only two blocks long, the Rue du Mont-Blanc had a lot crammed into it: a Protestant church (one of the few in a very Catholic country) at the foot of the street; an ordinary Belgian bakery at the corner that, to us, was a festival of freshly baked bread, croissants, pastries, and other goodies starting at 7 o'clock each morning; a Spanish butcher's shop across the street, hung with gigantic hams and other smoked meats; a bordello up the street that disgorged a steady stream of embarrassed men, hitching up their pants and scanning the street furtively to ensure that no friends were watching; and a grocery at the top of the street, whose young Italian owners made fresh pasta every afternoon. It was the sort of neighborhood where the children could go anywhere by themselves (although to my knowledge they never visited either the church or the bordello) without our having to worry about their safety. We had been warned that Belgian families were extremely insular, that we would be lucky to discover so much as the names of our neighbors. Instead, the family in the townhouse next to ours knocked on our door the day we arrived and brought us an apple tart from the corner bakery.

Even in pleasant surroundings, living in Belgium was more stressful than staying home. Belgians do everything a bit differently from Americans; that often turned the most routine chores into nerve-fraying adventures. The amplitude of my tremor was an accurate stress meter, and by that gauge, speaking French ranked high. The result was garbled communication. Soon after we arrived from Washington, I nervously asked a clerk at a dry goods store for charcoal; he led me to the shoe section. Judy didn't have any better luck. Once she noticed a strange reaction to her request at a kitchenware store for a replacement glass bowl for our coffee maker. Later she discovered that she had actually asked for a plate glass window.

The European style of banking also registered high on my tremor stress gauge. In Europe, I discovered too late, people hardly use checks at all. Instead, they pay bills by transferring funds electronically. It took me two weeks to set up procedures allowing me to make electronic transfers from the Los Angeles bank where my paycheck was deposited to my Belgian bank. In the meantime, we lived almost entirely on things we could buy with credit cards. Even after money transfer became routine, our troubles with the local banking system weren't over. In our first December, while I was out of town, Judy tried to use our bank debit card at a gas station one evening. But the machine rejected the card: insufficient funds. That was surprising because we had a line of credit of 100,000 Belgian francs—more than $3,000—and as far as Judy knew we hadn't used any of it. Only later did we learn that we had been undone by another feature of the Belgian banking system: automatic payment of utility bills. Until December, the gas and electric utility had estimated our energy consumption according to the pattern for the building's last occupants. When the building had been split into four flats, the tenants were all poor, and none used much gas or electricity. As a result, we paid hardly anything in our first few months. Then in December a meter reader visited the house. The subsequent bill, unknown to us at the time, exceeded $3,000! So that evening, Judy paid cash for just enough gasoline to limp home. For a few days—until we had unfrozen our account with an electronic money transfer from Los Angeles—Judy and the kids again lived on our credit cards.

Even when we could afford gasoline, driving meant stress. Most Brussels intersections are uncontrolled by either traffic lights or stop signs. In fact, there may not be more than a half-dozen stop signs in the city of a million people. Instead, the rule of the road is "priority to the right"—which means that you can gun it into the intersection as fast as you can as long as you don't hit somebody coming from your right, and if you hit somebody from the left, it's the other driver's fault because you had *priorité à droite.* I became so accustomed to this after three years that when I returned to Washington, I drove for many weeks with my head tilted to the right.

My tremor rarely deserted me during those early days in Brussels, but it was seldom incapacitating. My family has no memories of its interfering with any of our activities. In fact, the children, who have hardly known me any way except shaky, have few Parkinson's-related memories of Brussels at all. Margaret's is the one I like best. When she overheard one of Will's friends asking why his dad shook so much, she interrupted: "Don't make fun of my dad."

As for work, I decided to approach it as I had in Washington: by telling people immediately why I had a tremor and then dropping the subject. The first to receive this treatment were the candidates for my office assistant's job. I informed each that my disease might force me back to Washington before the end of my three-year rotation. None expressed any interest in dropping out of the competition. As a result, I had to choose among four or five extraordinarily well-qualified candidates. I made the right choice: Isabelle Maelcamp, a recent college graduate who felt stifled as an assistant to a Japanese journalist. She organized my professional life and turned out to be a reliable and resourceful reporter, and she provided further evidence that not all Belgians are unfriendly and standoffish.

For my first major assignment—a survey of the world economy—I went to London to meet some of the best minds in Europe's financial capital. My first in-person interview in Europe was with the chief economist of the brokerage house Morgan Stanley. Naturally, my tremor responded vigorously to the stress. As in the United States, I quickly explained my Parkinson's diagnosis. The economist reacted the same way that nearly everyone did: he offered his condolences and then moved on. In fact, the interview went so well that at the next one with a Goldman Sachs economist, I was completely steady and did not mention my health.

I took advantage of my trip across the English Channel to consult with an eminent British neurologist. I was leery about entrusting my health to a doctor in Belgium who had not grown up speaking my language, and Dr. Reich had steered me to Professor C. David Marsden.[1] While I waited in his office, Professor Marsden took the trouble to read the file that I had brought from Dr. Reich. Then he talked with me at some length about my options and concluded that I seemed to be doing everything about right. He probably spent half an hour with me, and as I left, his secretary presented me with the bill: 300 pounds (then about $600) payable in cash. As I howled in astonishment, she asked, "Oh, dear, did I forget to tell you that it might be a trifle expensive?" She certainly had: I didn't have enough money with me to pay and sent the final 100 pounds by mail. The reason for the exorbitant cost, I decided later, was the existence of a private health care system parallel to the British National Health Service. As part of the public system, Professor Marsden, like every physician in Great Britain, was paid a salary by the government to treat every British citizen who needed his services. Salaries are set at levels substantially below what doctors can earn in most other European countries, which in turn is much less than in the United States (where I used to think doctors were shamefully overpaid until my stepdaughter became one). But there was nothing to stop physicians from compensating with patients like me— patients who fell outside the British system—and those British citizens who were willing to pay extra for a higher degree of care.

My experience with Professor Marsden exposed another difference between the United States and Europe. A tension exists between the public's unlimited demand for medical care and the health care system's limited ability to provide it, and the tensions have been resolved differently on the two sides of the Atlantic. Europeans—and this is true on the continent as well as in Britain—have accepted less individual choice. The British health system controls costs by limiting doctors' salaries and openly rationing care. In Britain, patients go on waiting lists for operations from hip replacements to liver transplants, even if they may die before reaching the head of the line. On the continent, most countries rely on regional health-planning boards to add a little more flexibility to what is still rationed care. Either way, all citizens theoretically have equal access to the health care system. By contrast, the United States has abandoned the goal of universal access to top-flight health care. In our market-driven system, some 43 million Americans—about one in six—had no health insurance in 1999,[2] and these uninsured were unlikely to see a doctor until they wound up in a hospital emergency room. I'm inclined to favor the European approach as more civilized and equitable.

Certainly I grew comfortable with the Belgian health care system. Thanks to my stepdaughter, Theresa—who talked the George Washington University medical school into giving her academic credit for spending a month at a Brussels hospital—I found a neurologist who spoke better English than I did. The most striking thing about Dr. Diederik Zegers de Beyl was his full, dark beard. Otherwise, he was of moderate height and physically unimposing, but he certainly knew his stuff. For about $30 for a consultation in his office at the Erasmus Hospital (conveniently located at the end of one of Brussels' many tram lines), he guided me through the rest of my three years in Europe. His treatment philosophy matched Dr. Reich's: use enough medication to go about your business, but no more. He seemed particularly interested in Parkinson's surgery. When he asked me what operations were available at my hospital in the United States, I described one in which the surgeon kills a few brain cells to suppress tremor. He shook his head.

"In Europe," he told me, "that operation is considered to be practically cause for a malpractice suit. If the surgeon misses his target, he can make you blind instead of stopping your tremor." He recommended that I go instead to the university hospital in Grenoble, at the foot of the French Alps, where surgeons were suppressing tremor—without the danger of blindness—by implanting electrical stimulators in the brain. I soon spent the better part of an afternoon with Dr. Pierre Pollak, one of the world's pioneers in this operation. Although I felt far from desperate enough to want brain surgery, I asked if my disease was sufficiently advanced that I qualified for the operation. He tried to put a harness on me to measure the amplitude of my tremor. But (in Dr. DC's memorable phrase) I was shaking like anything, as I usually did when talking about my health. Dr. Pollak could not secure the harness. "Never mind," he said. "You qualify."

Such occasions aside, my tremor seldom ranked as more than an annoyance during my years in Europe. I conducted more interviews by phone than I would have without the tremor, although I generally prefer the phone anyway because it's quicker. When I interviewed in person, I tried to sit at a table or a desk instead of out in the open, where my vibrating legs would be visible. I used a tape recorder when my shaking reduced my handwriting—which is barely legible when I'm steady—to random squiggles. Whenever my tremor was conspicuous, I explained its cause. Like the Morgan Stanley economist, everyone accepted the explanation and said nothing more.

I had arrived in Europe taking only two mild anti-Parkinson's drugs. Artane, like the medication that Charcot used more than a century earlier, is a relative of belladonna and suppresses the tremor. And selegiline, then a brand new compound, was thought to slow the disease's progression. I also took a low dose of Mysoline, which reduces the familial tremor that I had inherited from my mother. In fact, the dose was so low—half of a 250-milligram tablet per day—that I couldn't imagine it had any effect. So I wasn't worried when I ran out of Mysoline just before flying to Geneva to cover a meeting of the Organization of Petroleum Exporting Countries (OPEC). On the plane, however, I shook so hard that I spilled soda all over myself, and I didn't even try to eat the dinner. This was one of the worst bouts of the shakes during my three years in Europe. The missing Mysoline was the only explanation I could think of. I was relieved to discover I didn't need a prescription to get Mysoline in Switzerland. I bought an emergency supply from a pharmacy, and my tremor subsided shortly after I took the first pill. Maybe it was just a colossal coincidence. But to this day I faithfully take a small daily dose of Mysoline at bedtime.

After a year overseas we returned briefly to Washington for Theresa's medical school graduation, and I went to see Dr. Reich. He and I agreed I had grown shaky enough that it was time to roll out the heavy artillery. He prescribed levodopa, which did a terrific job of blocking the tremor. When I took it, I looked no more as if I had Parkinson's disease than my dog did. After returning to Brussels, I discovered that I could actually use my laptop computer on, of all places, my lap. (Previously my legs couldn't hold the computer steady.) Along with the levodopa, Dr. Reich put me on yet another drug, called bromocriptine, whose chemical structure resembles the brain's missing dopamine. By fooling some brain cells into behaving as if it were the real McCoy, bromocriptine reduces the amount of levodopa necessary to control the tremor.

During my three years in Brussels, the levodopa usually performed superbly, although it took a little getting used to. One morning shortly after I began taking the medication, I was scheduled to interview the European Community's top trade official. Too rushed to have breakfast, I took my first pill on an empty stomach. Fifteen minutes later I threw up. Luckily the nausea faded quickly, and I was fine for the interview. That was the only time levodopa had that effect; my system quickly adjusted to the medication and did not try to expel it. At first a single blue pill, split in two, half swallowed in the morning and half in the late afternoon, kept me steady all day.[3] Over time, each dose opened a smaller window of steadiness, and it was not long before I needed to open my pill box three times a day and then four. Still, I was often fairly steady without levodopa. Typically, I could read in the peaceful pre-dawn hours without medication. I usually took my first levodopa about half an hour before driving the kids to school or going to work—thirty minutes being the time the medicine needed to make its journey to the brain.

One condition could disarm levodopa: extreme fatigue. At least with my regular dosage, the pills could no longer conquer the tremor when I was too tired. I spent a hectic month in Moscow in the fall of 1991, when the Soviet Union was disintegrating. Ten *Los Angeles Times* reporters had converged on Russia and the other republics that had composed the Soviet Union. My job was to be their editor, directing their movements and editing their stories. That meant starting the day around 9 or 10 o'clock in the morning—when the reporting began—and ending it at 3 or 4 the next morning, the deadline in Los Angeles (eleven hours behind Moscow). Luckily there were a few hours in the afternoon when the correspondents were reporting or writing and had not filed stories. That allowed me to hustle back to my hotel and take a nap that, along with a third half of a levodopa pill, kept me tremor-free through the night.

But on a couple of other occasions, there was no time for naps. I was one of three *Los Angeles Times* reporters in the Dutch town of Maastricht in December of 1991 for the signing of the treaty that created a single

European currency (the euro). The leaders of the twelve countries that then made up the European Community met late into the night of Tuesday, December 12, before announcing an agreement at nearly 2 o'clock the next morning. By then my ability to type had almost deserted me, and I had to dictate the lead of the next day's story to one of the other reporters. Because the East Coast newspapers' deadlines had passed, we were the only newspaper in the world whose correspondent reported the signing of the Maastricht treaty in all its Wednesday editions.

Again, in August of 1992, a European currency crisis brought many of the continent's financial officials to Brussels. Their key meeting went late into the night, but this time I had a plan. I asked Isabelle to wait outside the meeting room while I stayed home, popping an occasional levodopa tablet, writing the background sections of the next day's story, and preparing to include whatever information Isabelle could add. It was above and beyond the call of duty, but Isabelle cheerily stuck to her post until the sky began turning light at 5 A.M. At last the financial officials announced their decisions—the most significant were the devaluations of the British pound and the Italian lira—and Isabelle phoned. By then it was too late for the early edition in Los Angeles, but I sent the story in time for the home-delivery edition—another scoop, thanks to the time zones.

Except for these extraordinary events, Parkinson's hardly handicapped me in three years as the Brussels correspondent. My editors knew better than to send me to a war zone, such as Bosnia. But short of that, little was off limits. My most memorable assignments involved places rarely visited by Westerners. Atop my list was Trnava, a little town in Slovakia, which was then still part of Czechoslovakia. I was reporting a story on Eastern Europe's dangerous nuclear reactors, and Trnava had the closest hotel to an antiquated reactor at Bohunice. The hotel room was spare: little more than a mattress and pillow on a raised concrete slab, coarse sheets, a thin blanket, and a bare lightbulb in the ceiling. The price was about $2 a day, including dinner and breakfast. At dinner the beer was extra. When I couldn't surmount the language barrier to determine how much it cost, I tossed in 10 Austrian schillings, or nearly a dollar. The waiter was blown away by this huge sum of Western money. I could hear him and other waiters whooping it up in the kitchen, no doubt laughing at the stupid American who had paid a whole dollar for a bottle of beer.

I worked hard in Europe because that is the only way I know. But I was also determined to vindicate Shelby's decision to send a Parkinson's patient overseas. I sensed at the time that Shelby's move was exceptional. Not until I returned to Washington and joined a support group of young Parkinson's patients did I realize how exceptional—and courageous—his decision had been.

There was, for example, the sobering story of Larry McCurdy, a computer specialist who monitored information technology contracts for the Food and Drug Administration. Before Larry's Parkinson's days, his supervisors consistently gave him above-average evaluations. In 1996, his immediate boss wrote five memos praising his work. That year Larry (born thirteen days after me) noticed a mild tremor in his right hand. By year's end, a neurologist had diagnosed Parkinson's. Like me six years earlier, McCurdy couldn't suppress the symptoms, and like me, he notified his boss. That's where the similarities end. As Larry recalls, his boss—without so much as an "I'm sorry to hear the news"—seemed to go out of her way to compound Parkinson's misfortune. She downgraded his responsibilities and gave him assignments that preyed on his greatest weakness: writing longhand with his shaky right hand. As writing became all but impossible and even typing became hard, he asked for a laptop computer for taking notes in meetings and a voice-activated computer for his office. She responded by demanding a report from his doctor. When that justified his request, she asked for a second opinion. When it turned out the same as the first, she brought in an FDA doctor, who rejected McCurdy's claim as groundless. It was only in March of 1998, a month after his boss had moved to another job within the FDA, that he was given a voice-operated computer.

McCurdy's boss had a different take on events. She said she assigned projects to Larry that matched his abilities, which, she said, fell short of his pay grade after he developed his symptoms. Larry had not, she insisted, been "harassed, intimidated or demeaned."[4] Who is right, Larry or his boss? My reading is that both were right, from their own angles. To his bosses, Larry was an underachiever who used his disease as an excuse. But they certainly came up short in compassion for a man whose future was suddenly compromised. McCurdy didn't take it passively. He filed an equal employment opportunity grievance with the Health and Human Services Department, the FDA's parent agency. Vindicating Larry on his central complaint, the department judged that the length of time taken to provide him with his special equipment violated the 1973 federal Rehabilitation Act. In August of 2000, three and a half years after Larry had notified his boss about his Parkinson's, the department awarded him $5,000. As I write this, he is preparing to appeal to a jury for a larger award.

Then there's the case of Sandy Forney, who was a billings analyst with IBM when she got the news about Parkinson's in 1989. Her job also required much handwriting as she annotated billing records, and the disease, as it often does, made her handwriting progressively smaller and harder to read. She felt that IBM—like the FDA in McCurdy's case—went out of its way to give her assignments that emphasized her weaknesses, while disregarding her own suggestions to make the job more manageable. She proposed annotating the billing records with color-coded stickers instead of handwritten notes; the company, without explanation, said no. When driving to work became dangerous, the company—after lengthy delay—set her up with a home computer but insisted that she still commute to the office at least one day a week. In 1994 she participated in clinical trials of experimental Parkinson's treatments at the National Institutes of Health. As part of those trials she was subjected to two spinal taps, and the procedures sufficiently weakened her that she retired from IBM on disability benefits at the end of the year.

Some people with Parkinson's seem eager to leave their jobs and live on disability benefits, even when they could keep working. A friend of a colleague of mine in Los Angeles wouldn't discuss how she was doing on the advice of her lawyer, who warned that she could lose her disability benefits if it became known that levodopa (which she doesn't take for fear of potential side effects) could suppress most of her symptoms. But I most definitely would not put Arthur J. Cook Jr. in this category.

Art Cook, a patient of Dr. Reich's who lives near Baltimore, thinks his former employer, the Baltimore County Police Department, forced him to retire at age 47 from his job as lieutenant in charge of police training programs and may have caused his Parkinson's. Not long before Art began having difficulty walking, he and his co-workers noticed dead cockroaches in the old school building that served as their offices. They contacted the county pest control office, which had contracted with a private company to rid the building of bugs and said the contractor had sprayed pesticides only outside the building. Cook and his colleagues arranged for an independent testing firm to evaluate that claim. The day before the inspection was scheduled, a stranger equipped with heavy-duty cleaning equipment walked unannounced into the building and headed for one of the bathrooms. Art asked what he was doing. He replied that he had been instructed to clean the interior of the building thoroughly. When Art said any cleaning would be done over his dead body, the stranger left.

To this day, Art isn't sure who the man was or where he came from. But this much is certain: the independent tester arrived the next day and found "saturation levels" of four pesticides, including one so potent that it is supposed to be used only outdoors. Can pesticides cause Parkinson's? The jury is still out, although some studies have found a link. Can the symptoms follow the exposure as quickly as they must have in Cook's case? That's unclear. Regardless, his symptoms grew worse, and eventually the department suggested that he take his accumulated sick leave and try to recuperate. When his sick leave ran out, the department offered to place him on early retirement with disability benefits equal to half his salary. He thought about challenging the offer but then thought better of it: "It gets to the point where you can't fight city hall."

Art's story has a rare happy ending. A year after his retirement, he learned that Loyola College in Baltimore was looking for someone to train its forty campus police officers, just as he had trained the county police department's two thousand. When he was interviewed for the job, he could hide his Parkinson's symptoms at first; but the interview stretched over two hours, and by the end he was quite shaky. So he acknowledged having the disease and figured that would be the end of that. He was surprised when he was called back to a second interview, and astonished when he was offered the job. The pay isn't great, but with his disability benefits, he is earning as much as he did from Baltimore County. And Loyola, far from making his life difficult, lets him keep his own schedule; when he needs to take time off to see a doctor, there are no questions asked.

Art is surely one of the rare people who have found new jobs after contracting Parkinson's, just as I'm one of the few whose employer would consider sending them overseas for three years after the disease struck. I can understand why employers are wary of us. There is no denying that we gradually work more slowly and less efficiently. At some point, we can no longer pull our own weight. As I write this, eleven years from my diagnosis, I have surely slowed from the pace I maintained when I was in my early 40s. I think I'm still earning my salary, but sometimes I wonder. My sixtieth birthday—the benchmark I set when Dr. Reich diagnosed my Parkinson's at age 46—is now only about two years away. I fully intend to still be working then. But I won't be able to maintain my 1990 pace. And the chances of my staying at my current job until I'm eligible for Social Security retirement benefits (which will happen when I'm 66) are growing more remote. I might be able to improve my odds by undergoing one of the operations that relieve some of the more intrusive symptoms. And there's always the possibility that researchers will develop a cure just in the nick of time. But I want to be prepared, emotionally as well as financially, if I don't make it.

In My Doctors' Words
Professor C. David Marsden, London, October 1, 1990
(writing to Dr. Reich)

Many thanks for asking me to see this charming editor for the *Los Angeles Times,* who has had the misfortune to develop Parkinson's disease at an early age. . . . Luckily he has little functional disability although the tremor is quite severe. His walking is good without imbalance. Apart from difficulty with handwriting, manual skill is unimpaired for practical life. His speech and swallowing are normal. His general health is good, although he has lost some weight probably due to his Parkinson's disease. His memory is excellent.

For a period of childhood, he was subject to dizzy spells and had two episodes of loss of consciousness. Against a background of an abnormal EEG [electroencephalogram] these seemed to have been construed as epileptic, for he took diphenylhydantoin between the ages of 10 and 24. He has had no problem like this since. . . .

On his present drug regime the only possible side effect is occasional dizziness, although this is not a major problem. He also describes sweating spells, which I think are a part of his Parkinson's disease. The diagnosis of Parkinson's disease is secure. . . .

As to treatment, he is very well read and knows all the options. He has settled for delaying levodopa therapy until functional disability warrants it. He is coping very well on his present regime and I have not made any suggestions to change it. He is not keen on stereotactic surgery at this time.

We had a long talk about Parkinson's disease in general and I hope the consultation was of value to him. I have offered to see him at any time at his request during his stay in Europe over the next three years.

Dr. Steven G. Reich, Baltimore, May 28, 1991

From the standpoint of his activities of daily living, Mr. Havemann functions at a very good level, but this requires a great deal of effort.

It is particularly hard for him to take notes. He remains embarrassed and "awkward" due to the tremor, but fortunately, it does not impede his socialization. . . . He says that he tries not to think about Parkinson's disease, and just takes things "one day at a time." He is concerned about the effect Parkinson's may be having on his children, but so far, nothing adverse seems to have happened to them. He is having a very good experience in Brussels, and professionally, remains quite active. . . .

I don't think we are going to get much more mileage out of the medications he is currently on, and as a matter of fact, he has been intolerant of higher doses. As such, I think it would be prudent at this time to give Sinemet a trial.

Dr. Diederik Zegers de Beyl, Brussels, June 7, 1993

Mr. Havemann Joel was seen for the first time at my out-patient clinic in March 1991, when he was 47 years old. . . . When I first saw him the main problem was a rest tremor of the right side which was quite large and interfered with his daily life. Tremor would also appear when he kept the right arm outstretched after about 10 seconds. There was also rest tremor of the left lower limb. He also complained of some stiffness in the right shoulder and feeling dizzy when getting up.

The physical examination in June 1991 showed moderate bradykinesia [slowness of movement] of both arms, moderate rigidity at the right wrist and the right elbow, quite significant rest tremor of the right side and of both lower limbs, mild hypokinesia of the face [inability to make facial gestures] and hypophonia [soft voice]. . . .

Sinemet was introduced in July 1991. . . . Mr. Havemann thought that his improvement was significant and that even his rest tremor had improved by about 30 per cent. His handwriting was also easier. Orthostatic hypotension became worse. . . . Between July and November 1991, Parlodel (bromocriptine) was introduced at a moderate dose (8 mg/day). It did not significantly improve his condition.

In May 1992, after several months of progressive weight loss, the diagnosis of pulmonary tuberculosis was made and the patient was treated with an association of Rifampicin, Pyrazinamide and Isoniazid (INH). His parkinsonian condition deteriorated in a catastrophic manner after starting the anti-tuberculosis drugs. When INH was changed and replaced by Ethambutol, his condition somewhat improved. However, he was still much worse than he was before his anti-tuberculosis treatment. In order to help him continue his job during this time, . . . apomorphine was given as a nasal spray at the dose of three times 1.5 mg per day, and this has helped him during the first few weeks. Anti-tuberculosis drugs were stopped in December 1992, and his condition improved somewhat after that. . . .

He was able to cope with his job quite well and the tremor was his main handicap. . . . His handwriting was of quite poor quality, although I just managed to read it. He has some very mild hypophonia, and the speech was completely intelligible. Rising from a chair was quite easy. With walking, there was a diminished arm swing bilaterally, more so on the right with a slight tendency to scuff the right foot on the ground. His turning was quite easy, his posture was upright and there was no postural instability. Although the tremor was of quite variable amplitude from one visit to the other, when it is bad it tends to shake his entire body. . . . Because of the severity of this tremor, I suggested to him to see Dr. Pollak at the Centre Hospitalier Universitaire de Grenoble. Dr. Pollak saw Mr. Havemann in May 1993 and suggested that chronic stimulation of VIM [a part of the thalamus] was a good [strategy] to control his tremor. Mr. Havemann will think about this treatment in the future.

Dr. Pierre Pollak, Grenoble, May 7, 1993

One indication for bilateral thalamic stimulation is the severe handicap caused by the tremor. I explained how the operation would go. It is necessary to count on 15 to 20 days in the hospital. We didn't address the question of cost, but we have never had any problem with foreign patients; even in the United States, insurance companies pay the entire hospital charge (estimated at about 60,000 francs [$12,000], everything included).

CHAPTER FIVE

The Darkest Hour

It should be the function of medicine to help people
die young as late in life as possible.
— Ernst Wynder, president, American Health Foundation

BACK IN WASHINGTON after three years in Brussels, we picked
up our old lives as if we had never been away. We moved back into the
same house. The kids went back to the same school. Judy returned to
the *Washington Post* (although now as an editor, not a reporter). And I
slipped back into my old editor's slot in the *Los Angeles Times* bureau.

But I had new worries as I lay awake night after night, listening to the
cuckoo clock strike 4 in the morning. One was the very fact that I was
awake. Parkinson's disease takes its toll in many ways; the most devastating for me then was its refusal to allow more than four or five hours of
sleep. Once my medication had worn off, my tremor shook me awake.
No amount of counting by thirteens could put me back to sleep. At
work, I usually needed an afternoon nap; sometimes I would nod off at
my desk or, still worse, during meetings. When evening came I collapsed into bed, so exhausted that even the tremor seemed to have no
energy left. Within five hours or so the cycle began anew.

But by the last week of 1994, more immediate concerns intruded.
Almost two years earlier, while I was in Brussels, my mother died
suddenly in the suburban New Jersey home where I had grown up. One
minute she was climbing the stairs after breakfast; the next she was on
the floor, dead. Of my parents, she was the luckier. She died quickly and
painlessly. Dad had depended on her totally. They had few friends, and
days passed when they talked only to each other. Dad had always
assumed he would die first. He never expected to have to manage on his
own. I tried to reassure him by promising him that he could live with us
once we returned to Washington in about six months. He barely lasted.
When I arrived from Brussels, his house looked as if it had been overrun
by Sherman's march to the sea. Filth and garbage were everywhere—
some store-bought, some man-made. All available evidence pointed to a
steady diet of rum-raisin ice cream; nothing else seemed to have been
eaten.

A couple of weeks later, when we left the house for the last time, Dad didn't look back. He had lived there for forty-four years, more than half his life. During those years he had established himself as possibly the best magazine writer of his generation, traveled to the Soviet Union at the height of the Cold War, owned winning race horses, collected $61,908 on a $2 bet at a racetrack in Tijuana, Mexico, and written a trailblazing college psychology textbook. All this—and not even a backward glance.

It must have been 5 o'clock in the afternoon when we squeezed into Dad's tiny Hyundai to drive to Washington. At dinner along the New Jersey Turnpike, I blundered—although I didn't know it then—by ordering franks and beans. Beans are high in protein, which (I learned later) obstructs levodopa's journey from the intestine to the brain. Within half an hour, my tremor announced itself with the customary twitch in my right hand. After an hour, the shaking was uncontrollable. Driving the turnpike at night in a strange, small car is difficult enough when you're steady. If you're vibrating violently, it's almost suicidal. I swallowed levodopa tablets like candy. It made no difference. Dad, bless him, stayed cool. I stopped at every rest stop to stretch; never did he become impatient, though it was soon past his regular 10 o'clock bedtime. Before leaving I had thoughtfully placed several pipes and his humidor behind the front seat so that he could relax with a smoke. When he asked for his pipe, I proudly handed him one and, looking for tobacco, opened the humidor. No tobacco—the humidor had been used in the kitchen to hold bacon grease so that it wouldn't clog the drain.

I had finally just steadied down when we pulled up in front of our house in Chevy Chase at about 2 in the morning. Dad's basement apartment, the one our babysitter and her daughter had used before our years in Brussels, was ready—and he was ready for it. But once settled in, he spent most of his waking hours upstairs with the family. A loner all his life, he found that being entirely alone, without Mom, overwhelmed even him. Early every morning, before anyone else was awake except me, he would slowly drag himself up the twelve steps from the basement to the kitchen. I can still hear him grunting with every step.

Judy and I consciously decided not to shelter our children from old folks. But I don't know if the experience with Grandpa made them more or less compassionate. To those who didn't know him well, Dad was not an attractive person. Some of his habits—notably his addiction to his pipe and his insistence on a glass of 7-Up on ice at midmorning—drove the kids nuts. We hired a full-time housekeeper to watch Dad while Judy and I were at work, but that still left nights and weekends. The job wasn't difficult until he became incontinent, about a year and a half after his arrival.

Dad, as I've said, detested old age. He hated it in others, and he particularly hated it in himself. He would sooner have lost all his money at a racetrack than live in a nursing home. Ten years earlier he had written an eloquent letter, also signed by Mom, to their lawyer, their doctor, and Judy and me. They had just visited an old friend in a nursing home. "We come away from our visits consumed by pity for our friend," he wrote. "She was always high-spirited and feisty; now all the fight has gone out of her. She was extremely intelligent; now her child-like environment is eroding her judgment. We mourn too for her fellow sufferers at the home. What were they like when they were still themselves? Surely they were decent and lively people, now reduced to horrible caricatures."

Dad described nursing homes as "expensive tombs for the living dead." He pleaded that he and Mom be allowed to die—even be put to death—if they became nursing-home candidates: "True, the human spirit seems to cling to life of its own accord, blindly seeking to survive regardless of circumstances. Those people in nursing homes, lying in a coma, keep breathing for weeks and months and sometimes years. They are helpless and hopeless, yet their hearts still beat. The patients babbling in their wheelchairs are mentally dead, yet they remain physically alive. We too may fight death by reflex action. We may even, if we are speaking, say that we want to keep living forever. If we do, that will be only a sign of deterioration—something we would never have done if still in possession of our faculties."

By late 1994, Dad hadn't lost his mental powers, but his body was failing. Just after Christmas he fell in his apartment and painfully wrenched his back. Then he developed diarrhea and became dangerously dehydrated. On New Year's Eve, while the rest of the family left on a long-planned vacation, I stayed behind and checked Dad into a hospital. The nurses cleaned him up, got some liquids into him, and sent him home on January 2.

Back at the house, Dad grew progressively weaker. He couldn't walk. His world, which once reached from Tijuana to Moscow, shrank to the fifteen feet between his bed and his easy chair. He talked increasingly about having a "conversation" with his doctor, a code word for asking how he could bring on his own death. He never had to. That spring he caught pneumonia, which he refused to treat, ostensibly because the antibiotics would wreck his stomach. One morning, during my routine visit to get him up and give him a little breakfast, I found him choking on his own phlegm. I tried to sit him up. That made his breathing more difficult. I called 911. His heart briefly stopped as the ambulance arrived. The paramedics massaged his heart back into action, put him on a ventilator, and rushed him to the nearest hospital.

If I wanted Dad to die rather than to suffer, I learned later, calling 911 was a mistake. Many hospitals, once they receive a patient on a ventilator, refuse to turn it off. Luckily, Dad's hospital was not in this category. The emergency room doctor diligently explained what would probably happen if the ventilator was removed: Dad, unable to breathe for himself, would quickly die. As it happened, Dad had more gas in his tank than the doctor imagined. After removal of the ventilator, he didn't stop breathing until the next night, but he never regained consciousness, and—in my mind—he had died in my arms that morning.

Could I have prolonged his life by checking him into a hospital for his pneumonia? Probably. Would I have been doing him a favor? Hardly. Dad's mind had never stopped working. When he died, he was leading me in our annual backgammon tournament by thirty-two games to twenty-two. But if he had spent even a single night in a nursing home, he would have been acutely aware of his fate and deeply resentful. I feel some pride that he never did.

Dying has been much complicated by modern medicine's ability to keep us living far beyond what nature intended. We all fear death, but we are beginning to fear the last years of life even more. My parents were among the fortunate: Mom died in an instant; Dad's plunge into the abyss took only a day and a half. What were those thirty-six hours like for him? Was he at all conscious? Did he have any idea that he was dying? Could he hear what was going on around him? Did he hear me say I loved him?

How lucky I am that neither of my parents, lifelong smokers both, died of cancer. They did not have to endure the searing pain that ultimately consumes the body. In the 1970s, Stephen Rosenfeld, later the *Washington Post*'s editorial page editor and now a Parkinson's patient, wrote a moving book about how cancer killed his parents within seven months of each other.[1] What an ordeal—for parents and son. In the generation since, medical science has developed more ways of prolonging hopeless life. Shouldn't the final years be lived in dignity rather than humiliation and misery? None of us, no matter how powerful in our prime, are immune. As I write this chapter, Alzheimer's disease has reduced Ronald Reagan to a shell. Harry Truman, shortly after my memorable encounter with him in Kansas City, must have suffered a similar fate. David McCullough's biography, otherwise so thorough, virtually ends fully eight years short of Truman's death, when Truman falls in the bathroom, cracks his head against the washbasin, and breaks two ribs. After that, McCullough writes, Truman simply became "pitifully frail."[2]

We've become expert at caring for helpless individuals in the first year of their life. Medical science can snatch babies as small as a pound and a half from the grave. But we have hardly begun to think carefully and critically about life's last year. We should not treat the two as if they were the same. A newborn child has a whole life ahead. Medical intervention at that stage can yield benefits stretching over many decades. For the elderly at death's door, medicine pays no such dividends.

There are legal precautions you can take to avoid spending the end of your life helplessly and hopelessly attached to machines that breathe and digest your food for you. I learned of some of them at my thirty-fifth college reunion. When Harvard grads get together for a good time, they tend to go into classrooms and listen to each other conduct seminars. And once they're in their late 50s, the seminars include such old-age subjects as death and dementia. At one seminar, doctors and lawyers recommended signing a legal document—a "health proxy," as it is sometimes known, or "durable power of attorney"—authorizing someone else to make your decisions if you become incapacitated. Two oncologists said only a few of their terminal cancer patients had broached even the possibility of such a step. "Living wills" and other "advance directives," which spell out your desire to forgo "heroic measures" to prolong life, can also help. But because they can never address the precise circumstances that ultimately develop and the measures to be forgone, doctors and hospitals can ignore them—and frequently do.

A recent series of studies financed by the Robert Wood Johnson Foundation painted a disturbing picture of the last months of persons over 80 who are hospitalized and then die, either in the hospital or at home. Many of them—particularly cancer patients but others as well—endure great physical and emotional pain. The expense of keeping them alive often drains family savings. Surviving relatives frequently feel betrayed by the way hospitals make end-of-life treatment decisions that disregard patients' wishes.[3] Press accounts have vividly documented the consequences for patients and their families when living wills and other advance directives go unheeded. Particularly striking was the case of a public relations official with a New York cancer center, whose severely demented mother lived in a nursing home. Despite a living will, a health care proxy, and a keen awareness of the issues, the daughter could not shield her mother from unwanted hospitalization for a mild fever. "My poor, frightened mother was taken from her bed at night and brought by ambulance to a hospital," she said. "She was like an infant, in terror. She had a living will, prepared by an attorney, and I worked in health care. I had done lectures. I had handed living wills out to people. How come they didn't work?"[4]

Hospitals have at least two good answers. For one, they fear that living wills do not automatically protect them from legal action if their patients could have benefited from more intrusive care. And second, they stand to collect substantial payments from the insurers of their gravely ill patients. Their behavior will be difficult to change as long as these financial incentives remain in place. Although it seems cruel to say it, the enormous medical resources consumed by those in their final days and weeks leave that much less for medical care that would be welcome and might actually help.

Of course, these life-and-death issues are a moral swamp. Nobody has a crystal ball showing exactly when the last six months of life begin. Nobody wants to lean so far in favoring death over painful life that denying heroic medical care evolves into a tool for eliminating an unpopular mother-in-law. But surely we can improve upon the present balance. I am much more comfortable with the Dutch solution than our own. The Netherlands has legalized doctor-assisted suicide in carefully defined cases of "unbearable" physical or mental pain from an incurable condition. The doctor making this determination must know the patient well, and the first doctor's opinion must be certified by a second doctor and by a regional commission.

Let's now advance the calendar to the summer of 1999. On a typical evening, I'm editing *Los Angeles Times* stories on my home computer. Or at least I'm trying. Judy's 93-year-old mother, Lola McIntosh, won't give me a moment's peace. Although she sleeps in our house, she lives in a world created entirely by her imagination. Her memories are almost entirely false. But that makes them no less real to her.

"I want you to drive me home as soon as you can," she says as I try to ignore her and concentrate on a story. "Do you know where home is?

I think I'll get home. I think I will. My father [he died more than fifty years ago] gave me a good car. I haven't used it yet."

Does she have Alzheimer's disease? Almost surely, although there has been no formal diagnosis. Her behavior fits the standard descriptions: forgetting names and recent events, mixing reality and fantasy, becoming incontinent, wandering off, repeating things endlessly. Although she lives in her fantasy world, sometimes that world intersects with our own, almost by accident. One morning before anyone else in the house was awake, I was serving her a breakfast of crepes with strawberries and blueberries when she said, "It's nice to have somebody treat me like I was almost human."

In May of 1996, we had all traveled to northern Michigan to celebrate Grandma's ninetieth birthday. Then, she was sufficiently aware to understand and enjoy all the fuss. But over the next year she went noticeably downhill. She lived alone in a government-subsidized apartment building in a town near her old farm. Occasionally she walked out of the building and, when someone stopped her, explained that she was going to the farm—about ten miles away. In the spring of 1997, the management notified Judy that Grandma couldn't stay. So Judy flew to Michigan for her mother's ninety-first birthday, bundled her into her 1986 Ford, and drove her—it took three days—to her new home in the basement of a house on Woodley Road in Washington that we had bought the year before.

By the time Grandma arrived, her mind had permanently deserted her. Those readers of my age (born in 1943) may remember Art Linkletter, the TV personality, whose trademark phrase was "Kids say the darnedest things." Well, so do the very old. One afternoon I took Grandma to the hairdresser's. As we arrived back home, she thanked me and said pleasantly, "That was a nice trip. I hope you can stay for dinner."

Her tone was almost always cordial and calm; the effect was not. She lost track of time. She often slept during the day and remained awake at night. More than once she ate an early dinner, went to sleep for a few hours and woke up around 9 o'clock, wondering where breakfast was. As if Judy and I didn't have enough trouble sleeping, she made it harder. One morning just before 6, during one of those rare hours when Judy and I were both asleep, she walked quietly into our room and said triumphantly, "So this is where you sleep!" On another occasion, while I was sleeping on the living-room couch, she walked up to me quietly and said, "Are you sleepy?"

She was convinced that her mother was still alive—in fact, she regularly called Judy her mother—and falsely believed that her father had walked out on her mother soon after the birth of their only child. One day, when our mail included a solicitation for Alzheimer's research, Grandma said, "That might help my mother and father. They're alive, you know." By contrast, she never mentioned the man to whom she had been married for nearly forty years or the son who had died in a car crash in 1992.

It wasn't that she didn't like to talk. In fact, she talked and talked to any available adult, pursuing her prey throughout the house as if determined to prevent a moment's peace. Occasionally her ramblings made sense. Her sporadic reminiscences often focused on the first two or three years of her life. Born in Iowa, she suffered early from a nearly fatal bone infection around her eyes. (So primitive was medicine in the first decade of the twentieth century that the doctor treated the infection by making an incision in her eyebrow and scraping away the infected bone. A more painful process can hardly be imagined.) Despite her medical history, she yearned to return to her childhood; she regularly talked about her plan to drive back to Iowa. I took notes on one typical passage, which veered suddenly into incoherent fantasy:

"Where's your wife? [Judy was in Seattle at the time.] I didn't want to disturb her. She didn't think she was enough with that person to do a top job. I think different, but that's all right. I can be different. Are you ready to go with me? If you'd take me to my mother, that's the best you could do. The trouble is, she's too good. She wants to tell you what to do and how to do it. She was a schoolteacher. I want to call her to make sure she's there. I want to go where I used to go to school and to play."

Grandma's manner would have been funny if it weren't so sad. Her bad hearing and failing memory made her an almost impossible conversational partner. Once we took her with us to a party given by an Iranian-American couple. The wife's mother, Zaman, lived with them and spoke only Farsi. Well, the two women got into a long conversation. They were perfectly matched: Zaman couldn't understand what Grandma said and Grandma couldn't hear what Zaman said.

Dinner-table conversation at home also had its moments. Here's one conversation, shortly after Judy, Margaret, and Will had visited friends in New Jersey:

Judy: "It was so nice today to see Jan; she's just as much fun and as full of life as ever."

Joel: "What's their new house like?"

Grandma, pointing to Will: "That boy has a good appetite."

Judy: "It's a huge ranch house with five or six bedrooms on at least two acres of land."

Grandma, referring to her caretaker when Judy and I are at work: "That woman has an awfully large family. She took me to see them today."

Judy: "Yes, Mother. You've told us that five times already."

Grandma: "I have? Well, I'll be darned. My memory isn't so good any more, you know. After all, I'm more than 100 years old."

Judy, referring to Jan's daughter: "Liz has become a terrific swimmer, and she has medals and trophies all over her room."

Grandma: "You know, that boy has a good appetite."

Slowly, inexorably, Grandma wore us out. Marian, our housekeeper, was with her every weekday; we didn't leave her alone for a minute. But Marian worked only about 50 hours a week; that left us in charge for the other 118. We had to be on alert even in the middle of the night, because Grandma would regularly wander around the house—and beyond. One spring morning, Grandma was gone. I dashed outside and, unable to locate her, ran to the neighborhood police station, which luckily is only a couple of blocks away. To my relief, the first person I saw was Grandma, who was enjoying all the fuss being made over her. She had wandered two blocks from home to the busiest street in our neighborhood. Two passing joggers had seen her and, figuring that an old lady in a bathrobe didn't belong there at 6 o'clock in the morning, asked if they could take her home. Of course Grandma didn't know where home was, and so the joggers took her to the police station. After that, we installed "Grandma locks" on our doors—bolts that were too high for Grandma but within reach of the rest of us.

There was no escaping Grandma inside the house, a fact that exasperated Judy and me. I could manage Grandma better than Judy—Judy wouldn't disagree—because I was more patient and resourceful. I teased her, gently, in a way she found funny. When she insisted that she owned a white car parked in front of our house, I'd say: "Oh, that's not yours. You've always had fancier cars than that." When she couldn't find her shoes, I'd say: "No wonder, they're so small you can't see them." (She took a size 3, which she could find only in the children's department.) Judy could never invent these games. It's partly the difference in our personalities, but it's mostly the difference between being a child and a child-in-law. It's hard to be playful with someone who gave birth to you, nursed you, changed your diapers, and raised you. It was also hard because, now that Grandma needed to wear a diaper, Judy changed it, just as I'd changed my dad's diaper. (Was this a matter of gender or parentage? If it had been my mother, who would have had diaper duty? I think that gender controls—that Judy and not I would have been responsible for changing my mother—but I'm not sure.)

As with my father, we believed keeping Grandma with us could teach our children compassion. But here, too, the experience did not seem to inspire either tolerance or understanding. The children resented having to baby-sit for Grandma, as they often did, particularly between Marian's quitting time of 6:30 P.M. and our arrival home from work, typically an hour later. It upset them that Grandma couldn't remember their names—she called them, collectively, the Managers. (It was no consolation that she couldn't remember her own name either.) It bothered them that Grandma made the house smell funny, that she made a mess of her food at mealtime, and that she thought the dog was hers and not theirs.

Finally Judy and I began looking for somewhere else for Grandma. Our friends said we'd been heroes for hanging on so long, but we felt miserable. What we found was not exactly a nursing home. In the late 1990s, there was an explosion of "assisted-living" homes for the elderly who did not need round-the-clock nursing care but could not live on their own. With Alzheimer's patients alone estimated at four million, the demand for assisted-living units was practically limitless. We found a place we liked out in the foothills of Virginia's Blue Ridge Mountains. It was called, simply, The Home. All the authoritative guides gave it high marks, as did a reporter in my office whose mother lived there. We dreaded the day in the fall of 1999 when we finally packed Grandma into our station wagon and drove her to The Home. But Grandma inadvertently made it easier. While Judy filled out the paperwork, Grandma went into the dining room for lunch with other residents. Afterward, Judy asked if she had made some new friends. "Oh, no," Grandma responded. "I knew most of them already."

For a few months, Judy was content to visit on weekends. But the day before Thanksgiving, Marian drove down and brought Grandma back for the holiday. We knew Grandma wouldn't know she was missing anything if she remained at The Home, where the turkey-day dinner was spaghetti. We also figured she wouldn't have a very good time with us—and even if she did, she wouldn't remember it. Still, no matter how annoying Grandma could be, none of us could abide her spending the holiday eating spaghetti with strangers while we overate at Theresa's house in Baltimore. So when I returned from work on Wednesday, Grandma was sitting in her old familiar chair.

But it wasn't the old familiar Grandma. How weak she had become after only a couple of months of living away from us! She couldn't stand up unless somebody held her. Her legs had grown too weak to support even her small body, which had shrunk to seventy pounds. She had a terrible time getting food from plate to mouth. A scar down the middle of her forehead marked where she had cut herself falling out of bed. But for all that, her state remained "pleasantly confused." She still smiled at a tease, although as Judy pointed out, she might have been responding to the tone of my voice as much as the words. And once, feeling good after a sensational dinner, she actually addressed Judy by name— something she had hardly ever done while she was living with us.

Back at The Home, Grandma grew stronger for several months. During the winter, when nearly everyone at The Home, residents and staff alike, came down with the flu, Grandma stayed healthy. But that trend did not last. In the following summer, she broke her hip in a fall. A surgeon pinned her hip back together, but she could never again walk properly. That did not prevent her from trying, and as often as she managed to put her weight on her bad leg, she fell and injured herself. Judy drove the four hours' round-trip to visit nearly every weekend. Sometimes she found her mother in good spirits; sometimes she found her withdrawn and belligerent. But never, from shortly after that last Thanksgiving with us, did Grandma show that she recognized her own daughter.

As someone with Parkinson's, I inevitably wonder how long I'll survive and what the final years of my life will be like. So far, as I write these words, I've managed more than eleven years since my diagnosis. I am two years from my sixtieth birthday, the target I had blurted out when Dr. Reich diagnosed my condition. But I do not expect to live as long with Parkinson's as I would have lived without it. The medical establishment argues otherwise. Dr. Abraham Lieberman, medical director of the National Parkinson Foundation, says the introduction of levodopa in 1969 made it possible for patients who take their medication properly to live every bit as long as anyone else. No doubt that's true for any individual. But the evidence strongly suggests that as a group, people with Parkinson's do not live as long as a comparable group of people without the disease. In the most recent study I have found—and it agrees with those that preceded it—researchers in Sicily kept track of 59 Parkinson's patients of all ages and a control group of 118 persons without Parkinson's. After two and a half years, 20 percent of the people with Parkinson's had died, but fewer than 10 percent of the control group had. The results were the same for the study's full eight years.[5] Dr. Lieberman argues that the Sicilian Parkinson's patients probably did not enjoy access to levodopa and other potent Parkinson's medications. In fact, however, the Italian researchers isolated the data on the Parkinson's patients who were taking levodopa. Death did not come to this group as fast as it did to those without levodopa, but it still came faster than to those without Parkinson's.[6]

People do not die of Parkinson's the way they die of heart attacks and cancer. Only a rare death certificate lists Parkinson's as the cause. But Parkinson's increases the vulnerability to other afflictions. Jim Backus, the actor who played Thurston Howell III in the 1960s television series *Gilligan's Island* and who was the voice of the cartoon character Mr. Magoo, died at 76 of pneumonia. He contracted pneumonia because Parkinson's had caused him to swallow some food down his windpipe into his lungs, where it became a breeding ground for germs. Sid Dorros, author of an insightful and inspirational book about life with Parkinson's,[7] died of septic shock resulting from constipation caused by the disease. At 76, Congressman Morris Udall died of the lingering effects of a fall down the stairs at home nine years earlier. The fall occurred because Parkinson's had robbed him of balance.

So I cannot avoid contemplating my own death. Nor can I know how I will react when my condition deteriorates seriously. But I do know that I fundamentally agree with my father and mother, whose letter I regard as an elegant statement of common sense: "Our society, at least until recently, has seemed determined to postpone death as long as possible, no matter how hopelessly the individual has deteriorated physically or mentally or both, or how expensive the effort. We have never understood why. Aging and death are simply the natural order of things— unstoppable and irreversible, as much a part of life as birth. We accept the inevitability without resentment and have no desire to fight it."

In My Doctors' Words
Dr. Stephen G. Reich, October 17, 1994

Joel returns today for reevaluation of young-onset Parkinson's, as well as familial essential tremor of the upper limbs. He feels that there has been no change since the last visit, and for the most part he is getting along well and remains active and completely competent with his activities of daily living. Emotionally, he is doing well, and his general health has been unremarkable.

Dr. Reich, October 9, 1995

He is doing very well and has had no significant problems since last visit. He is functioning at a good level, although he occasionally does have "tough moments." Psychologically, he is doing well, and his general health has been stable. He is experiencing some mild motor fluctuations with predictable end-of-dose wearing off but no dyskinesias and, for the most part, these are tolerable. He is very sensitive to dietary protein and conserves it throughout the day.

Dr. Reich, October 2, 1996

Joel generally looks well. There is diminished facial expression, and his voice is a bit soft, but perfectly intelligible. There is an intermittent resting tremor of the right hand, and mild cogwheel rigidity of the right upper extremity, but no significant bradykinesia. He walks well, and his posture is upright with no postural instability.

CHAPTER SIX

Today's Drugs

Medicine, to produce health, has to examine disease,
and music, to create harmony, must investigate discord.
—Plutarch, *Lives*

THERE IS STILL NO CURE for Parkinson's disease, and we can easily grow impatient with what appears to be the slow pace of progress toward discovering one. But things could be a lot worse—and, until recently, they were. If I had been born thirty years earlier and my Parkinson's had been diagnosed in 1960 instead of 1990, I would have faced a truly bleak future. Then, the most effective anti-Parkinson's drug was a relative of the medication that Charcot had used a century earlier in Paris. Our understanding of the disease had advanced only slightly, and the ability to treat it had advanced hardly at all. Without sedation, I would have shaken from morning until night. As it is, I take five kinds of medication daily. They do not cure Parkinson's, nor do they halt its progression. But for some years, they suppress the symptoms for much of each day. The result is to spare me and thousands of others from total dependency. We can enjoy lives that, if not entirely normal, are still productive and fulfilling.

The development of these drugs is the story of modern medicine: clever, sometimes brilliant (and sometimes lucky) breakthroughs that point toward potential applications, followed by a lot of hard slogging to turn the potential into reality. Science has conquered many infectious diseases because Alexander Fleming noticed that a mold contaminating a laboratory dish full of bacteria seemed to kill the bacteria. That not only led to his discovery of penicillin but also pointed researchers toward developing (after much painstaking work) other antibiotics effective against bacteria that penicillin did not kill. Anti-Parkinson's drugs follow this pattern. The basic discoveries leading to today's medications were essentially in place by 1960. Yet it took almost a decade for drugs to become commercially available. During that period, researchers in universities, hospitals, and, ultimately, drug companies did a prodigious amount of work.

Levodopa

The initial research that led, directly or indirectly, to all the new anti-Parkinson's medicines occurred mostly in Europe. In 1951, the Swedish pharmacologist Arvid Carlsson (engaged in research that won the Nobel Prize in physiology or medicine in 2000) identified dopamine among the many chemicals that scientists were discovering in the brain. Its function was at first unknown, and researchers struggled to figure it out. My particular hero is Oleh Hornykiewicz, a Ukrainian who was trained at the University of Vienna in the chaotic days immediately after World War II, then received a fellowship to Oxford in the mid-1950s. After Hornykiewicz returned to Vienna in 1958, his British tutor gave him a piece of advice: "Oleh, you should stick to dopamine—dopamine has a bright future." That was an invitation to do basic research—no one knew what dopamine did—and Hornykiewicz accepted it. Back in Vienna, he came upon two recent discoveries by Carlsson and other Swedish researchers. In the first, they found that a drug causing Parkinson-like symptoms in laboratory rats left the rats' brains depleted of dopamine. In the second, the dopamine in a dog's brain was found to be concentrated in the striatum, a part of the brain that helps govern movement. Putting two and two together, Hornykiewicz promptly performed autopsies on people who had had Parkinson's and found severe dopamine shortages. That was in 1959. "The brain dopamine deficiency in Parkinson's disease, today standard textbook knowledge, more often than not stated as a self-evident fact that needs no reference to the original observation—at that moment I literally could see it with my own naked eye," Hornykiewicz wrote later.[1] The research performed by Hornykiewicz, and subsequently extended by many other neurologists of the same era, made possible the development of the medications that keep me functioning today. The trouble was that the discovery did not automatically lead to pills.

The obvious cure for Parkinson's would be a drug containing an artificial supply of the dopamine that the substantia nigra can no longer produce naturally. When you swallowed the pill, the dopamine would be absorbed from the stomach or the intestine into the bloodstream, which would carry it to the brain. But it's not so easy to tinker with the brain's chemistry. One major obstacle is the "blood-brain barrier." The blood vessels that supply the brain end in capillaries so tightly packed that many big, complex molecules can't get through. The brain has evolved in this way for good reason. The most delicate of the body's organs, the brain needs a stable environment in which to function; it can't afford the equivalent of hot dry weather one day and a snowstorm the next. In addition, unlike the rest of the body, the brain has no white blood cells to fight infection, and even a minor invasion by a virus or a bacterium can do immense damage. Unfortunately, the blood-brain barrier also blocks many chemicals that could perform useful work if only they could cross into the brain. One of these chemicals is dopamine. (See figure 6.1.)

The brain's raw material for manufacturing dopamine, the amino acid tyrosine, easily crosses from the blood into the brain. There is no shortage of tyrosine in the Parkinson's brain; the problem is converting the available supply to dopamine. Transforming tyrosine into dopamine is a two-stage process. First tyrosine becomes L-dopa, or levodopa; then levodopa is converted into dopamine.[2] As it happens, even the Parkinson's brain, at least at first, can easily turn levodopa into dopamine. When 80 percent of the substantia nigra's neurons are dead or dying, the remaining 20 percent still have what it takes to manufacture enough dopamine. The problem in Parkinson's is that, despite the ready availability of tyrosine, the brain no longer has the proper equipment to turn enough of it into levodopa. What if the brain could be supplied artificially with levodopa? It is the good fortune of everyone with Parkinson's disease that levodopa *can* squeeze through the blood-brain barrier. And, again, the Parkinson's brain, at least at first, has no trouble converting levodopa into dopamine. So a supply of levodopa seems to be just what's needed.

We know this now, but we did not know it in the early 1950s. At about the same time that Hornykiewicz made his critical discoveries about dopamine, Carlsson and two other Swedish researchers found that levodopa, unlike dopamine, could cross the blood-brain barrier and breathe life back into tranquilized rats.[3] Hornykiewicz, deducing that levodopa was being converted into dopamine in the rats' brains, wondered whether the brains of people with Parkinson's could duplicate the feat. So he entrusted his entire supply of levodopa—all of two grams— to Walther Birkmayer, a neurologist at Vienna's Municipal Home for the Aged.[4] Following Hornykiewicz's instructions, Birkmayer (unhindered by the sort of regulations that now govern the human testing of new drugs) injected a levodopa solution into the veins of some Parkinson's patients at the home. The results, as recounted by the two scientists, were stunning: "The effect of a single i.v. [intravenous] administration

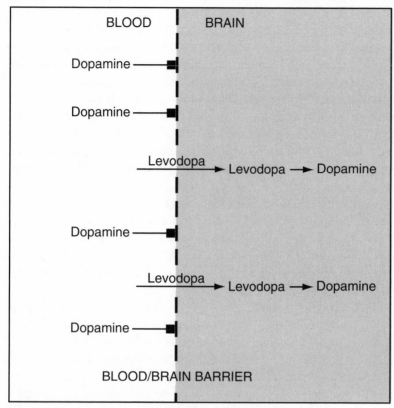

Figure 6.1. Dopamine cannot cross the blood-brain barrier, but levodopa can, and in the brain it is converted to dopamine.

of L-dopa was, shortly speaking, a complete abolition or substantial relief. . . . Bedridden patients who were unable to sit up, patients who could not stand up from a sitting position, and patients who, when standing, could not start walking, performed all these activities after L-dopa with ease. They walked around with normal associated movements and they could even run and jump. The voiceless speech . . . became forceful and clear again like in a normal person."[5]

This finding triggered a burst of research aimed at producing a pill for the mass market. For much of the 1960s, however, other studies failed to confirm Hornykiewicz and Birkmayer's finding. George Cotzias, a doctor at Brookhaven National Laboratory in New York, thought he knew why: Parkinson's patients were not receiving enough of the drug to do any good, because large enough doses made them vomit. Remember, Birkmayer had injected his precious supply of levodopa directly into the bloodstream of Parkinson's patients, which meant the levodopa bypassed the stomach. But this was not a practical way to administer levodopa to the masses. Cotzias got the idea of testing a way to avoid the vomiting caused by large oral doses of levodopa: building up a person's tolerance to it by starting with small doses and slowly increasing them. He tried this in sixteen patients. In 1967, he found that half of the patients showed "complete, sustained disappearance or marked amelioration of their individual manifestations of Parkinsonism." This was a huge breakthrough.[6]

Much work remained before levodopa could begin alleviating Parkinson's symptoms. Acquiring a tolerance to large doses of levodopa seemed to work for half of Parkinson's patients, but what about the other half? And that was just one challenge. Getting the levodopa from the mouth to the substantia nigra posed a major delivery problem. Perils and obstacles abound along the way.

The first is the stomach. Levodopa taken just after a meal sits in the stomach instead of proceeding to where it is needed. And even after it moves on to the intestine, levodopa must get into the bloodstream. It can't penetrate the intestinal wall on its own; it needs to be escorted by a special chemical that acts as a molecular taxi service. Although scientists don't fully understand this process, they do know that there's usually a waiting line for taxis. Amino acids, the building blocks of proteins, use the same taxis as levodopa and try to muscle their way to the head of the line. (See figure 6.2.)

I find that once I've eaten a protein-rich meal, any subsequent levodopa doesn't do me much good. So I eat practically no protein until dinner, when I'll be going to bed soon and won't need medication. I skip breakfast and, for lunch, eat a gargantuan fruit salad: apples, pears, bananas, kiwi fruit, red and green grapes, all kinds of melons—and, in the summer, plums, apricots, and even occasionally a few blackberries. All this largely protein-free fruit I store in the office refrigerator. If I have to go out for a working lunch, I usually order a cheese-free, meat-free salad—fruit if possible, green if necessary. I stay away from the fish, meat, or even pasta that people around me are eating. It's not always easy. Some years ago I attended a Parkinson's symposium at a local hotel. The morning's last speaker was Dr. Jonathan Pincus, a Georgetown University neurologist. Dr. Pincus, who is one of the world's

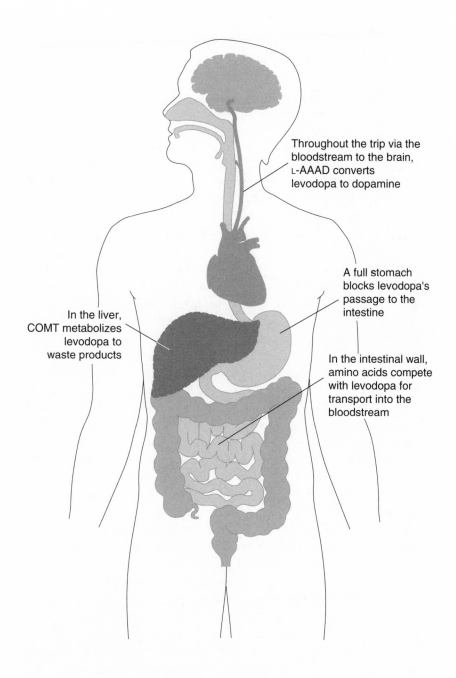

Figure 6.2. Levodopa, swallowed as a pill, faces a host of perils and obstacles on its way from the stomach to the brain.

leading exponents of the protein-free diet, talked about how most Parkinson's patients could live full, largely symptom-free lives if only they'd shun protein. So what lunch did the hotel serve to a room full of people with Parkinson's? Protein-rich tuna sandwiches!

Once in the bloodstream, levodopa encounters an enzyme named L-AAAD. In the substantia nigra, L-AAAD performs the essential function of converting levodopa to dopamine. Unfortunately, it does the same thing in the bloodstream, and levodopa does no good if it becomes dopamine outside the brain. Not only can dopamine not get through the blood-brain barrier but, to make matters worse, it stimulates the body's vomiting center, which is located just outside the blood-brain barrier. This explains the vomiting of Parkinson's patients who took large doses of levodopa.

The answer, in theory, was clear: to supplement levodopa with a compound that would block the action of L-AAAD in the rest of the body—but not in the brain. Drug companies saw the promise of an enormous market. Hoffman–La Roche, a Swiss pharmaceutical manufacturer, began experimenting with such compounds in the early 1960s. After Cotzias's 1967 study, academic researchers joined the chase. Birkmayer had good success with the compound benserazide; on the other side of the Atlantic, Cotzias did the same with a quite different substance, carbidopa. Hoffman–La Roche combined levodopa and benserazide into a single medication called Madopar, which became commercially available in Europe in 1973. Hoffman–La Roche also pursued the Canadian market. Dr. Harold Mars, a neurologist in Cleveland for most of his life, was working on Parkinson's in Montreal in the late 1960s (his father had the disease). At that time the only source of levodopa was a Japanese company that extracted the drug from the fava bean, a particularly rich source. Dr. Mars remembers receiving levodopa as one-kilogram bottles of white powder; he and his wife often stayed up late putting the powder into capsules that were given in huge quantities to Parkinson's patients, including his father.

At first the large doses sickened almost everybody who took them. Hoffman–La Roche soon introduced the same combination of levodopa and benserazide in Canada that worked so well in Europe. Dr. Mars switched to that medication, and his father was able to live the last five years of his life in considerably more comfort than he had spent the previous ten. Dr. Mars meanwhile went to Cleveland, but Hoffman–La Roche shunned the U.S. market because of the rigorous and expensive regulatory requirements of the Food and Drug Administration. With the

Medications Commonly Used to Treat Parkinson's Disease

Type	Brand Name	Generic Name	Usual Daily Dose	Mechanism	Adverse Effects
Dopamine precursor	Sinemet	Carbidopa/ levodopa	400–1,000 mg/day	Levodopa is converted in the brain to dopamine; carbidopa protects levodopa during its trip from the gut to the brain	Dyskinesias, low blood pressure, nausea, psychiatric disturbances
Dopamine agonists	Parlodel	Bromocriptine	7.5–30 mg/day	Mimics dopamine's action in the brain	Dyskinesias, dizziness, lethargy, low blood pressure, psychiatric problems
	Permax	Pergolide	2–6 mg/day	Same	Same
	Mirapex	Pramipexole	1.5–4.5 mg/day	Same	Same
	Requip	Ropinirole	3–24 mg/day	Same	Same
COMT inhibitors	Tasmar	Tolcapone	200 mg, three times per day	Neutralizes COMT, which attacks levodopa in the bloodstream	Diarrhea, dizziness, nausea, hallucinations, possibly fatal liver damage
	Comtan	Entacapone	up to 1.6 g/day	Same	Diarrhea, dizziness, nausea, hallucinations
MAO-B inhibitor	Eldepryl	Selegiline	5–10 mg/day	Neutralizes MAO-B, which attacks dopamine in the brain	Insomnia, confusion
Anti-cholinergics	Artane	Trihex-yphenidyl	2–10 mg/day	Restores the balance between dopamine and acetylcholine by blocking some acetylcholine in the brain	Confusion, dizziness, blurred vision, dry mouth, urinary retention
	Cogentin	Benztropine	0.5–6 mg/day	Same	Same
Other	Symmetrel	Amantadine	200–300 mg/day	Uncertain	Confusion, hallucinations, kidney damage

gigantic U.S. market wide open, the drug maker Merck, Sharp & Dohme offered a combination of levodopa and the compound carbidopa. It called the medication Sinemet, from the Latin words for "without" and "vomiting."

Even unimpeded by a stomach full of protein, levodopa can't travel from mouth to brain in much less than half an hour. And even with a carbidopa bodyguard, no more than one levodopa molecule of every hundred in Sinemet—and probably much less—gets to the desired destination. Each half Sinemet pill that I take contains 125 milligrams of levodopa. With luck, perhaps 1 milligram is converted into dopamine in the brain.

While levodopa is the strongest anti-Parkinson's drug, it has plenty of helpers that either enhance its effectiveness or complement its effects. My experience with these pills has been that they tantalized with early benefits but lost effectiveness within months. They enabled me to cut back briefly on my daily levodopa intake, but I soon had to beat a retreat back to where I had been. But who knows? Maybe these new drugs at least enabled me to hold the line instead of losing ground.

Dopamine Agonists

The dopamine agonists complement levodopa. They have a molecular shape so similar to dopamine's that they can lock into the same receptors. (See figure 6.3.) When I began taking levodopa in 1991, Dr. Reich also prescribed bromocriptine (brand name Parlodel), then the only drug of this sort in widespread use. I presume that the bromocriptine reduced the amount of levodopa I had to take. The drug companies worked overtime to produce better dopamine agonists. I switched first to pergolide (Permax), which for a few months was more effective than bromocriptine, and then to pramipexole (Mirapex), which was better yet.

The agonists are varied because the brain's dopamine receptors are diverse. The nerve cells that serve as dopamine receptors are of two basic kinds: those that are stimulated by dopamine and those that are inhibited. And within each type there is further variation: researchers have identified two distinct receptor cells that are turned on by dopamine and three that are turned off. Each agonist has a different combination of effects on the receptor cells. Which agonist works best for any individual patient? That depends on which receptor cells are particularly deprived of dopamine. The only way to find out is to try all the agonists to see which works best.

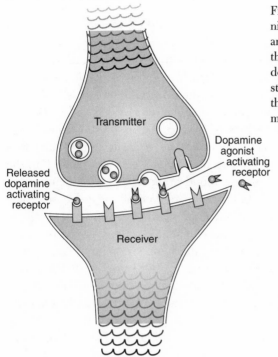

Figure 6.3. Dopamine agonists are so close in size and shape to dopamine that they fool some dopamine receptors in the striatum into thinking that they are actually dopamine.

COMT Inhibitors

Another set of drugs enhances levodopa's effectiveness, reducing the necessary daily dose. I've already described one of them. Carbidopa, the other ingredient (along with levodopa) in Sinemet, blocks the enzyme that converts levodopa into dopamine in the bloodstream, where it is useless because it cannot cross the blood-brain barrier. My newest drug, called entacapone (Comtan), is one of two now available to attack another enzyme in the bloodstream, called COMT.[7] COMT, which is found in particularly high concentrations in the liver, breaks down levodopa into its waste products (see figure 6.2). Entacapone's purpose is to prolong the action of each Sinemet pill and allow users to take fewer of them. For me, it initially cut my average day's intake of Sinemet from six and a half pills to five and a half. Is that worth the trouble? I think so; I faithfully swallow an entacapone pill (a big one that is difficult for someone with Parkinson's to swallow) six times a day. But as I write this, more than a year after I started taking entacapone, my average daily dosage of Sinemet has crept inexorably upward to six and a half or seven pills.

Selegiline

The surviving levodopa molecules that find their way to the substantia nigra are quickly transformed to dopamine, which carries messages to the striatum. Each dopamine molecule stands a good chance of returning safely back to the substantia nigra, where it is available for another trip. But maybe on one trip in five, the dopamine molecule has a fatal encounter with one of two predator enzymes, MAO-B and COMT. If only dopamine could somehow be protected from these villains, imagine how much more effective it would be. Well, it can, at least to a degree, from one of them. Entacapone, which combats COMT in the bloodstream, doesn't cross the blood-brain barrier and hence can't protect dopamine in the brain. But another of my pills, selegiline (Eldepryl), inhibits MAO-B in the brain. The FDA approved selegiline shortly before my Parkinson's was diagnosed in 1990. At the time, the drug promised not only to protect the brain's dopamine but also to retard the substantia nigra's deterioration. But selegiline has not lived up to that promise. I cut my intake of selegiline from two pills a day to one, but I found that going to zero set me back. Presumably the drug safeguards some dopamine.

Even this doesn't exhaust my daily regimen of anti-Parkinson's drugs.

Anticholinergics (Acetylcholine Inhibitors)

I still take a small amount of Artane (trihexyphenidyl), a close relative of what Charcot used. Before Sinemet in 1969, Artane and several related drugs were the only ones available. They inhibit the action of another of the neurotransmitters, acetylcholine. The message transmitted by acetylcholine is sometimes the opposite of the one carried by dopamine. Some of the consequences of too little dopamine can be offset by suppressing the effects of acetylcholine and restoring the balance between the two.

Amantadine

There is one common anti-Parkinson's drug that I've never taken. Doctors accidentally discovered that amantadine (Symmetrel), which was developed to ward off the flu virus, reduces Parkinson's symptoms for many people in the early stage of the disease. No one knows exactly why, but some of my friends say amantadine helped them postpone the day when they became dependent on Sinemet.

All this medication is expensive. The five anti-Parkinson's pills I now take cost $16.90 a day at drugstore.com.[8] That's $507 a month and $6,168 a year. But if drugs cost a lot, it's not simply because the drug companies want to stay highly profitable. American pharmaceutical manufacturers figure it takes twelve to fifteen years to develop a drug. That's a long time—long enough for something to make the drug obsolete before it gets to market. Parkinson's illustrates the problem. Novartis, the drug company that marketed Comtan (the brand name for entacapone) at the end of the 1990s, had been developing this drug for years. What if (horrors!) somebody finds a cure for the disease in the next couple of years? Then Novartis will have produced a very costly white elephant.

Every year the drug manufacturers invest some $20 billion in research and development—or somewhere between $300 million and $500 million for each new drug. The cost of bringing any one drug to market is far less, but for each success there are many failures. Perhaps a thousand or more compounds undergo preliminary screening but are discarded somewhere along the line as unsafe or ineffective. To allow the drug companies to recoup their costs, U.S. patent law protects new drugs from competition for twenty years from the date of the patent application. Only after the twenty years are up may other companies duplicate the chemical as a generic version of the original brand-name drug. For years, the brand-name drug makers had complained that the FDA was taking too much time—time during which the twenty-year clock was ticking—to approve drugs for sale. So in 1992, Congress passed a law enabling the FDA to accelerate the approval process with six hundred additional reviewers—reviewers paid for by the drug industry itself! That has speeded up the drug approval process, all right, but it has also contributed to some cases in which consumers died or became severely incapacitated after taking unsafe drugs, because corners were cut in the drug approval process.[9] What's more, the drug companies have not been content with the extra months or years of patent protection created by the 1992 law. They have found ways to extend the effective lives of their patents beyond the basic twenty years by, for example, paying generic drug companies to keep their copycat drugs off the market.[10]

Of my present five Parkinson's medications, three are brand names and two are generics.[11] Fortunately, my health insurance covers my entire $16.90-a-day habit. I sometimes worry about what will happen when—assuming I live that long—I retire and come under Medicare. Medicare does not now cover prescription drugs, although some members of Congress agree that it should and are pressing legislation to make Medicare do just that. But, at this writing, they have yet to decide how to pay for what would be a very costly new benefit. Naturally, I hope the stalemate is resolved. I don't look forward to paying out of my own pocket, as so many Parkinson's patients do now.

Drug companies and academic researchers have strived mightily to develop drugs to treat Parkinson's cardinal symptoms. But many of Parkinson's other symptoms have been virtually ignored. Researchers have given little specialized attention to constipation and difficulties in swallowing, for example, even though both have potentially fatal complications. Only recently has medical science begun to score some successes in the battle against Parkinson's mental effects, which are almost always drug-related. Levodopa, so effective against the tremor, does nothing for mental deterioration except sometimes enhance it. And the most widely used antipsychotic drugs aggravate some of Parkinson's physical symptoms.[12] Researchers have developed a new line of antipsychotic drugs that are less likely to enhance the movement difficulties of Parkinson's disease. With considerable success in many cases, doctors now often prescribe the drugs clozapine (Clozaril) and quetiapine (Seroquel) for Parkinson's-induced psychosis.

In medical laboratories all over the United States and in many other countries, researchers are looking for new anti-Parkinson's drugs that will improve levodopa's effectiveness. I wish them luck. But I hope their discoveries will prove of only fleeting value. A cure for Parkinson's is what all of us with the disease wish for: not a therapy that merely masks the symptoms temporarily but one that restores the brain to something like its original health. There's no telling how far in the future a cure lies. To bridge the gap between now and that wonderful day, medical science has developed surgeries that can help control Parkinson's symptoms when the medications have done all they can do.

CHAPTER SEVEN

Today's Surgeries

Surgery is always second best. If you can do something else, it's better.
—Dr. John Kirklin, heart surgeon, Mayo Clinic

THERE'S AN OLD CLICHÉ—a favorite of my dad's—to describe
something unwelcome, say, a flat tire or a bad cold: "I need that like a
hole in the head." Well, a hole in the head is precisely what I may
someday need. For many people, probably including me, levodopa's
side effects will eventually become intolerable. When that happens, the
next best choice is often brain surgery. In fact, before levodopa became
widely available at the end of the 1960s, surgery was the only Parkinson's treatment that was even moderately effective. It fell out of favor
when levodopa initially appeared capable of controlling Parkinson's
permanently. But once levodopa's limits and side effects emerged, surgery made a comeback.

Despite the obvious dangers of poking around inside the skull, brain
surgery has an astonishingly long and intriguing past—before written
history. Archaeologists have found evidence of cranial surgery in the
preserved skulls of human fossils thousands of years old. Stone Age
surgeons used primitive tools of flint and bone to remove pieces of skull.
The operation, now called trephination, seems to have served one of
two purposes, and sometimes both: to open an escape route for demons
that were thought to have entered the head and caused disease and to
relieve the pressure that was presumed to sustain bad headaches.[1]

Brain surgery barely advanced from the Stone Age until about 1900.
Then medical science began the remarkable series of advances that
improved its safety and effectiveness. Dr. Harvey Cushing, a neurosurgeon at Johns Hopkins in the first decade of the century, introduced
surgical techniques that made it possible to treat everything from headaches to brain tumors. Among his innovations were tourniquets and
clips to stop bleeding during surgery. Brain tumors were neurosur-
geons' principal target, and before Cushing, most attempts to remove
them killed the patients. In 1909, for the first time, Cushing successfully
removed brain tumors from more than twice as many of his patients as
died on his operating table.

Removing tumors was one thing; they were usually big and easy to find. Repairing parts of the brain that weren't functioning properly required a more sophisticated understanding of how the brain worked. Surgeons had to know what parts of the brain performed what jobs— and then to reach unhealthy spots without damaging nearby brain structures. Physicians had no answers early in the twentieth century. But that didn't stop them from trying. Because of a lack of effective medications, desperate patients would try almost anything. During the post–World War I encephalitis epidemic, Parkinson's was widely regarded as one effect of the encephalitis virus. Surgeons removed parts of the nervous system—notably in the spinal cord and the brain itself—that seemed likely places to harbor the deadly bug. Not surprisingly, many patients died as a result of the operation, and none were cured.

By the 1930s, physicians had located the part of the brain that wielded overall control of movement. They could reduce the Parkinson's tremor by destroying some of the cells in this area—but always at the cost of major inability to move at all. Trial and error led them to seek other neural circuits that, if interrupted, would relieve Parkinson's symptoms without such a devastating loss. By the mid-1940s, they were still searching for more precise techniques to navigate through the brain. The critical breakthrough came from two surgeons at Temple University Medical School in Philadelphia, Ernest A. Spiegel and Henry T. Wycis. But they probably couldn't have done it without the foundation laid four decades earlier by one of the odd couples of medical science.

In the first decade of the twentieth century, Victor Horsley, a British neurosurgeon, collaborated with Robert Henry Clarke, a mathematician, to build an apparatus that enabled them to study and measure a monkey's brain by holding its head steady. The apparatus consisted of a metal frame that was bolted firmly onto the monkey's skull. The frame looked a little like the superstructure of a crown, its spaces unfilled by fabric. Unfortunately, the two men fell out when Clarke wanted to apply the method to humans but Horsley scoffed at the idea as unrealistic. Each kept half the frame, which was useless without the other half. Horsley was especially headstrong. He convinced himself that heatstroke was an imagined condition that could not afflict the psychologically fit. Visiting Egypt in 1916, he insisted on working in the midday sun. He died of heatstroke.

Three decades later, Spiegel and Wycis collaborated more productively. Spiegel fled from prewar Vienna and was offered a research position at Temple. There he recruited Wycis, a young resident who earned his way through school by playing semiprofessional baseball and poker. Over the next twenty years, they studied Parkinson's and other movement disorders, as well as epilepsy, cancer, and pain.

Their major achievement came in 1947, when they developed a frame for the human head that made precise surgery possible. By then, X-rays enabled physicians to see a few landmarks inside the brain after injecting air into the brain's cavities, which ordinarily held only liquid. Having located the brain's landmarks, surgeons operated on other sites based on estimates of how far they were from the landmarks in a typical brain. That method, remembers Dr. Philip L. Gildenberg—a beginning medical student in 1956 who studied with Spiegel and Wycis for thirteen years—had two significant drawbacks. "For one, it caused a tremendous headache. We'd inject the air on a Tuesday, but the patient was too sick to have the operation until Thursday." And second, the distance from the brain's visible landmarks to the surgeon's target depended on the patient. "There's some variation in brain anatomy between individuals, just as some people have big noses and some people have small ones," said Gildenberg, a professor of surgery at the Baylor College of Medicine in Houston. Despite that, the Spiegel-Wycis frame had an enormous impact. Before it became available, nearly one patient in six died following surgery aimed at alleviating their Parkinson's symptoms. Spiegel and Wycis reported a mortality rate of only 1 in 50, and it soon fell to less than 1 in 100.

Once Spiegel and Wycis created their frame, the use of brain surgery exploded. Surgeons around the world adapted the new technique, called "stereotactic surgery,"[2] to old problems, including anxiety, aggressive behavior, epilepsy, and other convulsive disorders. Parkinson's disease—without any effective medication—got ample attention and benefited from some lucky mistakes. Dr. Irving Cooper, a renowned neurosurgeon, once accidentally interrupted the flow of an important artery in the brain during Parkinson's brain surgery. The patient, to Cooper's astonishment, awoke with no tremor. Cooper tried the same technique in other Parkinson's patients, with checkered success. He reasoned that the same artery fed different parts of the brain in different people. Ultimately he found that the interrupted blood affected the thalamus, a part of the brain that had not yet been associated with Parkinson's. From this developed one of the Parkinson's operations available today. This and other current surgeries all work on the same principle: that Parkinson's symptoms on one side of the body can be reduced by shorting out some of the brain's malfunctioning circuits on the other side. The globus pallidus and the thalamus are prominent in these circuits. Surgeons have found they can relieve some Parkinson's symptoms by burning out some of the cells in these two parts of the brain. Thalamotomy reduces or even eliminates tremor, but it has no effect on Parkinson's other symptoms. Pallidotomy is not as good at controlling tremor, but it often alleviates stiffness, slow movement, and dyskinesias caused by levodopa and other Parkinson's drugs. (For a schematic look at how pallidotomy restores one circuit to something like its proper balance, see figure 7.1, A and B.)

Today's surgeons still use a frame to steady the skull. Local anesthetics numb the areas where the frame is bolted to the skull and the spot—usually high on the forehead behind the hairline—where the surgeons insert their probe. They need the patient awake and responding so that they can tell exactly where to burn out some brain cells. The brain is chockablock with nerve cells, but luckily, they are not the type that registers pain. So once the probe is inside the skull, its further penetration through the brain is painless. Surgeons typically choose the quickest and safest route to the target inside the brain. "Generally you want to avoid veins and arteries," explained Dr. Roy A. Bakay of the Chicago Institute of Neurosurgery. "Some surgeons steer around the ventricle [the liquid-filled cavity within the brain], but we go through it." The route is programmed into a computer that already contains detailed information about the patient's brain from an MRI. Then the computer directs a tiny wire probe, much thinner than a silk thread, to the target. (A human hand, even one not afflicted with Parkinson's, would not be steady enough.) When the probe has reached its destination, the surgeon runs enough electrical current through it to temporarily deactivate the surrounding neurons. If the patient's Parkinson's symptoms do not respond, the surgeon moves the probe a millimeter or two until they do. The doctor then heats the probe sufficiently to destroy a ball of cells that, according to Dr. Bakay, is somewhere between a grape and a cherry in size. Dr. Bakay worries that, with so much of the procedure becoming computerized, the surgeon may become mostly a bystander.

But to the patients, the operation is hardly routine. It is often their last hope for relief from Parkinson's symptoms, and if something goes wrong, the result can be (but seldom is) death. Sandra Pollock was diagnosed with Parkinson's in 1986, when she was only 36. Her brand of the disease was marked more by slow movement and postural instability than by tremor. She had to quit her job as a special education teacher eight years after the diagnosis. Within ten years, the side effects of levodopa were almost as bad as the disease itself: "I couldn't hold a fork, and each limb was always going in its own direction. I just wanted relief." The best bet at the time looked like a pallidotomy. She met with Dr. Frederick Lenz, a Johns Hopkins neurosurgeon, and checked into the hospital on July 2, 1996. Here is her oral account of what happened.

That night they gave me a battery of memory and psychological tests, nothing more than that. The next morning at 7 they took me down to the basement in a wheelchair—I wasn't on a gurney yet. They had put a catheter in me because I wasn't allowed to eat anything. It was in the basement that they put the frame on me. It was square, not round like a halo, and it was made of metal. They secured it with two thumbscrews on either side of my forehead and two screws in back. They didn't pierce the skin, but they were tight. They had to be, because if the frame didn't hold my head completely still for the operation, the doctors might target the wrong brain cells. Then they made me lie down, and they strapped my head and neck down and did a scan of my head. They went inch by inch; it must have taken an hour and a half.

Then at about 10 they took me up to the operating room. It was very cold, I remember. For some reason I also remember that it was an all-male staff that was waiting for me. I was lying down on my back, and they gave me lots of pillows, but I still wasn't what you would call comfortable. My back hurt. But for the next four hours, there was no way I could move. It wasn't Dr. Lenz who was at the controls—it was somebody who seemed to be his first assistant. They spent most of the time trying to line up the microelectrode so that it would take out exactly the cells they wanted. It was all done by computer, and more than half way into the four hours, the computer went down. I panicked: would I have to come back and start all over? But after 10 minutes the computer came back up, and nothing seemed to have been lost.

Some time after that there was a lot of commotion behind me, and I briefly heard the sound of a drill. I couldn't actually feel anything, but they were drilling a hole in my skull so that they could insert the electrode. Later they gave me six stitches to close the cut they had made in my skin before they used the

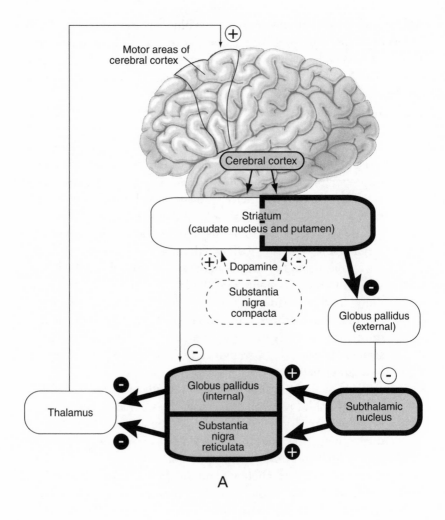

Figure 7.1. *A,* Because of insufficient dopamine, the brain of a person with Parkinson's disease does not effectively transmit messages. *B,* In a pallidotomy, the surgeon kills some cells in the globus pallidus. This has the effect of reducing the inhibition of the thalamus and, consequently, increasing the thalamus's activation of the cerebral cortex.

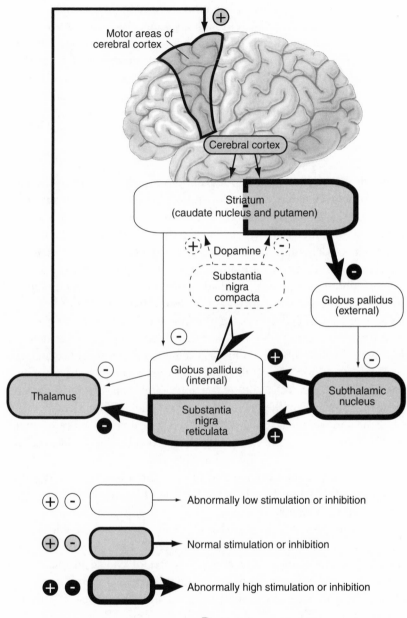

Motor areas of cerebral cortex

$\oplus$

Cerebral cortex

Striatum
(caudate nucleus and putamen)

$\oplus$ Dopamine $\ominus$

Substantia
nigra
compacta

$\ominus$

Globus pallidus
(external)

$\ominus$

$\ominus$

Globus pallidus
(internal)

$\oplus$

Thalamus

Substantia
nigra
reticulata

Subthalamic
nucleus

$\ominus$

$\oplus$

$\oplus$ $\ominus$ ⟶ Abnormally low stimulation or inhibition

$\oplus$ $\ominus$ ⟶ Normal stimulation or inhibition

$\oplus$ $\ominus$ ⟶ Abnormally high stimulation or inhibition

B

drill. When they finally used the electrode on my brain, I didn't feel any instant relief, although Dr. Lenz was by my side testing my arm to see how it responded, and he seemed very satisfied. In the recovery room I was seated in a comfortable chair, and they finally gave me something to drink. I got up to go to the bathroom, and I dropped something. I bent down to pick it up and straightened up again. I didn't think twice about it, but my husband was amazed. It was the first time in months that I'd been able to do that without falling.

Sandy was an ideal patient for a pallidotomy. The American Academy of Neurology recommends the operation for those who go suddenly from steady to shaky (so-called on-off fluctuations) and who experience disabling involuntary movements, called dyskinesias, as a result of levodopa. An academy task force found that patients in their 40s generally fared better from the operation than those in their 60s and 70s.[3]

Ed Calhoon was 54 when he had a pallidotomy at Johns Hopkins in 1997. Diagnosed seven years earlier, he found that the periods when his levodopa was ineffective were lengthening and that his dyskinesias were worsening. Dr. Lenz, who also performed Ed's operation, burned out four areas of the globus pallidus. Ed remembers the sounds generated by Dr. Lenz: "First I heard the drill motor start, then a loud crunching sound through my skull as he cut the hole." That was "the most anxiety-arousing moment" of the operation, Ed said later, with understatement. "It came and went in an instant, and there were no problems after that." As Dr. Lenz applied the heat to the targeted cells, Ed (unlike Sandy) immediately felt some of his symptoms disappear. Shortly after the operation, he resumed driving and playing the tuba. "The change has been dramatic," he said. "The operation is not for everyone, but for me it has been miraculous."

Nina King, the *Washington Post*'s former book review editor, was also 54 when she had a pallidotomy. She went to Sweden rather than get on the years-long line at her surgical center of choice in the United States, Emory University in Atlanta. She was ten years into the disease, and levodopa's side effects had eclipsed the disease itself. "It's the Catch-22 of Parkinson's," she wrote in the *Post*: "Enough L-dopa to quell tremor is enough to set off the side-effects. I was particularly bothered by L-dopa-induced 'dyskinesias': involuntary movements of legs, arms and head I dubbed 'writhing,' a friend called 'squirminess' and my mother described as 'flailing about.' Typically, I began the day very stiff, walked with a lurch, found it difficult to sit still for any length of time, had problems putting on a coat or pulling on pantyhose, and expended so much energy in involuntary movements that I would sometimes break out in a sweat sitting quietly at my desk. I also lost weight (10 pounds out of a 'normal' 110), and I felt exhausted a great deal of the time."[4]

Nina, like Ed, noticed her symptoms vanishing right in the operating room: "There was no tremor, no dyskinesia, and no rigidity." Her face, which had begun to sag, instantly looked better. "The only thing wrong with my pallidotomy is that its good effects did not last long enough," Nina wrote. "After about a year the symptoms began to return—gradually at first, more rapidly recently. It is now three years since my surgery and as I write this, I am writhing in a distinctly pre-op fashion." After writing that, Nina began to lose energy, and her sense of balance deserted her. Then she fell from bed and gashed her head. After the fall, she spent a week in a hospital and two months in an assisted-living facility. "I fell again at the rehab center, and falling is now my biggest fear," she told me in her new apartment a few months later.

"You look very good to me," I said. "Judy had warned me to expect the worst."

"I'm okay now [about half an hour before noon], but I go downhill after lunch," Nina said. "I figure I'm good for four hours in the morning. The rest of the day I try to keep from vegging." When I last called her, she was exploring the possibility of an operation on the other side of her brain. As she had written in the *Post*: "Have Parkinson's, will travel."

The deterioration that Nina experienced after her operation seemed to be greater than average. Surgeons at the highly regarded Parkinson's center at Emory, including Dr. Bakay (who moved to Chicago in 2000), found that pallidotomy's improvements remained significant four years after surgery. Although they admitted their sample of ten patients was small, they reported that tremor on the side opposite the operation remained nearly nonexistent. Other symptoms, while worse than immediately after surgery, were much reduced compared with before.[5] Surgeons at the University of Toronto found similar results.[6]

Pallidotomy's close surgical relative is thalamotomy. Doctors shift their sights slightly and destroy some cells in the thalamus, which is downstream from the substantia nigra. The actor Michael J. Fox had this operation seven years after his diagnosis in 1991, and it prolonged his television career by two years.

Thalamotomy generally works better than pallidotomy against

tremor,[7] but that is the only symptom it combats. When I was diagnosed with Parkinson's in 1990, Dr. Reich urged me to consider thalamotomy as a way of eliminating the tremor on my right side, then my only significant symptom. I held back, hoping for better treatments and fearing—correctly—that a thalamotomy might make it impossible to take advantage of them when they appeared. My tremor wasn't so severe that I felt compelled to take desperate measures. Besides, thalamotomy (and pallidotomy as well) is performed safely only on one side of the brain to relieve symptoms on the body's opposite side. When surgeons operate on the second side, slurred speech is a common side effect. If a thalamotomy stopped my right side from shaking, I wondered what I would do when the tremor spread to the left side, as it inevitably would.

In the late 1990s, a new operation—deep brain stimulation—seemed to disarm the dilemma. Instead of killing brain cells, surgeons implant electrodes in roughly the same places. The electrodes serve the same purpose—short-circuiting the brain's natural flows of electricity—without killing any cells. As a result, pallidotomy and thalamotomy are gradually giving way to the new procedure. The implanted electrodes are attached to a wire that runs down the neck and into the upper chest, all under the skin. The wire connects with a battery-driven pacemaker—the size of a pack of cigarettes—implanted under the collarbone. (See figure 7.2.) When the pacemaker delivers an electrical impulse, the electrodes block the brain's nearby neural pathways. The patient, by passing a magnet over the pacemaker, can turn it to high, low, or off.

This was the operation that, as Dr. Zegers de Beyl told me in 1993, had virtually made thalamotomy grounds for malpractice suits in Europe. It had taken so long to cross the Atlantic because of the Food and Drug Administration's painstaking approval process for new medical devices. In fact, when the FDA finally sanctioned the devices, it gave its blessing to performing the operation only at the thalamus. This meant that while doctors could implant the devices anywhere, Medicare and other government insurance programs would not pay for its implantation anywhere other than the thalamus. But many doctors performed deep brain stimulation at other locations anyway, for those who had other means of paying.

Although it is too early to measure the long-term effects, deep brain stimulation seems superior to pallidotomy and thalamotomy. "It's not a miracle by any means, but it's a tremendous advance," said Dr. Bakay. "It's safer and more effective than the older operations." A study in the Netherlands found deep brain stimulation of the thalamus to suppress

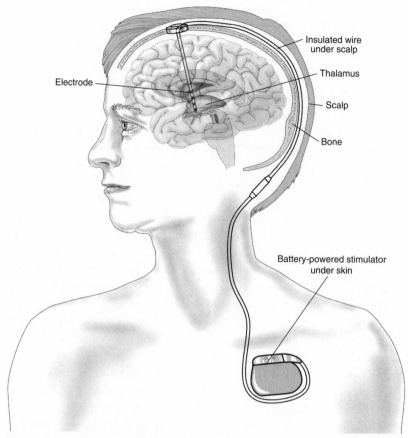

Insulated wire
under scalp

Thalamus

Electrode

Scalp

Bone

Battery-powered stimulator
under skin

Figure 7.2. In deep brain stimulation, electrodes are implanted in a strategic part of the brain (in this case, the thalamus) and are connected by a wire running under the skin to a battery-powered pacemaker placed under the collarbone. The electrodes can be turned high, low, or off by a magnet passed over the pacemaker. When the electrodes are on, they render nearby nerve cells inactive.

tremor as well as did thalamotomy, with fewer adverse side effects.[8] A more recent study found substantial improvements in muscle control for 134 patients on three continents who underwent deep brain stimulation. Patients who had typically been able to move normally for about one-quarter of their waking hours before the operation could do so for three-quarters afterward. They also needed less levodopa and had less of a problem with dyskinesias. Researchers declared deep brain stimulation more effective than pallidotomy, thalamotomy, and even fetal tissue transplants.[9]

Because deep brain stimulation leaves brain cells intact, it can be reversed if better treatments become available. It can be performed safely on both sides of the brain. And the patient, simply by passing a magnet over the pacemaker, can control the amount of relief delivered by the electrode inside the brain. Like any brain surgery, however, deep brain stimulation is dangerous. During the operation itself, patients run the risk of bleeding and stroke; one of the patients in the Dutch study died of a stroke. Short of that, the hazards of deep brain stimulation include infections where the electrodes, wire, and pacemaker are inserted. Paralysis and partial loss of vision are also possible. The pacemaker runs on a battery that has to be replaced, surgically, every three years or so.

When the electrodes are implanted in the globus pallidus, deep brain stimulation is the equivalent of pallidotomy. Likewise with the thalamus. But there is a third structure in the brain, called the subthalamic nucleus, where deep brain stimulation seems still more effective. Surgeons never destroy cells in the subthalamic nucleus because the risks are too great. But applying deep brain stimulation to the subthalamic nucleus was found in the multicontinent study to be highly effective and no more dangerous than implanting the electrodes in the globus pallidus or the thalamus.

The same French research center that pioneered deep brain stimulation found that using the subthalamic nucleus enabled many people with advanced Parkinson's to live independently again. Levodopa dosages could be cut in half, reducing the incidence of dyskinesias. But the French study found that bad side effects were also more common; one patient suffered severe paralysis and memory loss.[10]

Deep brain stimulation is the operation of choice for many people who have already had a thalamotomy or pallidotomy on one side of their brain and cannot risk the hazards of repeating it on the other side. Four years after the pallidotomy on the left side of her brain relieved Sandy Pollock's symptoms on the right side of her body, the disease had inexorably spread to her left side. Sandy, left-handed, grew concerned. She scheduled a deep brain stimulation for October 2000. It turned out to be quite an ordeal.

She had to be awake for the first part of the operation, when the surgeons implanted the electrodes in her brain. "It was pretty scary," she told me later. "When they were working on my brain I heard so many different sounds, like they were scraping out my skull with an ice cream scoop. That part of the operation took over six hours, and I had to be off my pills the whole time. I was reaching the end of my patience and my endurance. I was ready to cry."

By the time the electrodes were in place, Sandy had lost the ability to speak, and she had no feeling on her left side. That lasted for only about half an hour, she said, but her doctors, worried that she might have had a stroke, postponed the second half of the operation and admitted her to the intensive care unit, even though a CAT scan had revealed no sign of a stroke. She went home two days later and returned to the hospital in another six weeks to have the electrode connected by wire to a pacemaker implanted under her collarbone—a procedure performed while the patient is under general anesthesia.

"I do feel much better since the operation," she said. "I'm more smooth in my movements, not so rigid and taut as before. I have more stamina and feel more focused. I don't regret it, I guess, although the second operation was a lot more unpleasant than the pallidotomy."

Deep brain stimulation had just become available when Mike Kushnick (diagnosed with Parkinson's in 1981 at age 48) underwent the operation in 1999, and doctors were still resorting to trial and error. Surgeons at Johns Hopkins initially scheduled him for a pallidotomy. But his own neurologist, uncomfortable with an irreversible operation, sent him to the University of Virginia, which had begun offering deep brain stimulation. There, surgeons began exploring in his globus pallidus for the most effective place to locate the electrode. When they could not adequately tame Mike's tremor, they tried the subthalamic nucleus and had more luck. Mike remembers relaxing on the operating table as the surgeons hit the right spot.

He also remembers suffering one of deep brain stimulation's common side effects—hallucinations. "For five days I thought that people were taking me up and down in an airplane, that the Chinese cavalry was charging me. I had to be tied down to keep from running away." The cause of the hallucinations is not known, although Mike's doctor told him that it might result from too much air entering the cranial cavity during the operation. In any case, the hallucinations usually go away in a few days—and, fortunately for Mike, this was the case with him. A year after his operation, Mike showed no sign of his old tremor, although he needed a considerable amount of levodopa—one full gram a day—to suppress it. His chief visible symptom was slow movement.

To me, the amazing thing is not that these procedures work so well but that they work at all—that they can be performed with a high degree of confidence that the patient is not going to die on the operating table.

Altogether, surgeons now perform a million operations a year on the nervous system, the spinal cord as well as the brain. The overall death rate in 1998 was about 5 percent, and even that figure is swollen by stroke patients who fail to survive their emergency surgery.[11] For thalamotomy, pallidotomy, and deep brain stimulation, the death rate is substantially under 1 percent. One researcher surveyed the results of thalamotomies in the 1980s and found a death rate of less than three patients in a thousand—generally from bleeding in the brain or a postoperative infection.[12] This is so even though the government, which carefully screens drugs and medical devices before allowing them to be sold, exercises no such control over surgical procedures. All it takes for an operation is a combination of a desperate patient and a willing surgeon.

What surprises me under these circumstances is that so few people with Parkinson's undergo operations each year. Reliable statistics don't exist, but the National Center for Health Statistics has counted only about 2,500 thalamotomies, pallidotomies, and deep brain stimulations a year in recent years. Professionals who deal with Parkinson's patients every day say less than 10 percent of them qualify for the operations; the rest are too old, have symptoms that resist surgery, or otherwise do not make suitable candidates. But that still leaves as many as 100,000 candidates for the operation. Maybe, as the literature suggests, those of us with Parkinson's really are a conservative, risk-averse lot. Most apparently view surgery as I do: as a last resort that, while statistically safe, is a frightening prospect. I'm still not signing up for the next open date at the Johns Hopkins neurological operating room. But it's reassuring to know that if my pills fail me, as seems almost inevitable sooner or later, another, surprisingly safe form of relief is available.

CHAPTER EIGHT

An Insidious Beast

Hitherto the patient will have experienced but little inconvenience; and befriended by the strong influence of habitual endurance, would perhaps seldom think of his being the subject of disease, except when reminded of it by the unsteadiness of his hand, whilst writing or employing himself in any nicer kind of manipulation. But as the disease proceeds, similar employments are accomplished with considerable difficulty, the hand failing to answer with exactness to the dictates of the will. Walking becomes a task which cannot be performed without considerable attention. The legs are not raised to that height, or with that promptitude which the will directs, so that the utmost care is necessary to prevent frequent falls.

—James Parkinson, *An Essay on the Shaking Palsy*

NOW ELEVEN YEARS since my Parkinson's diagnosis, I still regard my pills as enough to keep me healthy. When they are working—which is most of the time—I'm steady and relaxed. My fingers sweep across the computer keys as effortlessly as when I was half this age. When I run into old friends who haven't seen me for a while, they often comment on how healthy I look. That's a tribute to my drugs, particularly levodopa. Without them, I would be a trembling cripple twenty-four hours a day.

Instead, as for everyone else on levodopa, my physical condition has three states: underdosed, just right, and overdosed. Underdosed is where I am in the early morning, before my first levodopa pill kicks my shakes away. Just right is where I want to be, with enough levodopa being transformed into enough dopamine to make me feel normal. Overdosed is where I frequently wind up, squirming and writhing and lurching because too much dopamine is swimming in my synapses. For most of the day, I can still keep myself just right if I balance my intake of medicine and food carefully. If my friends catch me then, they have trouble spotting my disease. But the proper balance is growing harder and harder to achieve because there are fewer and fewer surviving nerve cells in the substantia nigra to regulate the brain's dopamine level.

When my dopamine level dips too low, my symptoms grow more

severe. Although the tremor is my most obvious symptom in the under-dosed condition, I display all the cardinal signs of Parkinson's to one degree or another. My muscles, particularly those of my trembling legs and arms, are flexed and rigid.[1] I move at about half my former speed—a condition known medically as bradykinesia. And my posture deterio-rates: I bend at the knees and the waist, giving me a hunched-over look. In this state, once-routine tasks become difficult, and once-difficult ones become impossible.

My first concessions to the disease seemed trivial. When the tremor made shaving with a blade dangerous, I switched to an electric razor. Cutting my nails became impossible in my "off" state, which meant not doing it first thing in the morning, as I always had. I couldn't rotate my hand to flip pancakes, beat eggs, or brush my teeth until I had pro-gressed from "off" to "on." I couldn't even shake things effectively; Parkinson's shakes are not the same ones needed to shake an orange juice carton. Gradually the disease's victories grew. I gave up playing tennis; the last time I tried, I tripped over my own right foot. I won't climb more than three rungs up on a ladder, for fear of falling. Because I can go from steady to shaky between freeway exits, I gave up driving more than a few miles on busy highways without someone who can jump into the driver's seat. At each of these retreats, I have sworn to make a stand the next time. But so far, the disease has always prevailed.

Being hyper is better than being "off"—but not much better. My nonstop squirming probably bothers those around me more than it does me. But my balance is worse when I have too much dopamine than when I have too little. My walking style is slow and zigzagged. It's easier to run than to walk—sometimes I have to run just to keep my feet under my center of gravity. I lurch from place to place like someone in a funhouse where the floor is tilted one way but appears tilted another. I'm sometimes mistaken for drunk, although my problem is surplus dopamine, not alcohol. In a healthy brain, there are enough nerve cells in the substantia nigra to store dopamine until it is needed to cross a synapse. In my brain, the nerve cells in the substantia nigra are too few to perform this regulatory role.

These movement and posture problems were only Parkinson's ad-vance guard. Like a rancid smell that slowly fills a room, the disease eventually interferes with many aspects of physical and mental well-being. There are two reasons. For one, dopamine governs the proper functioning of much more than arm and leg muscles. For example, it also affects the autonomic nervous system. Operating largely subconsciously, this part of the nervous system controls such bodily functions as digestion and sexual response. The second reason is that Parkinson's attacks regions of the brain other than the dopamine-producing substantia nigra. These other regions govern a variety of mental and physical activities. No wonder Parkinson's disease affects different people so differently: its pattern of nerve cell destruction varies widely from one person to the next.

During my early office visits with my neurologists, Dr. Reich and Dr. Zegers de Beyl, they always asked, "Do you show any signs of impotence? How about incontinence?" For a year or two I confidently laughed at the questions. Surely that couldn't happen to someone as young as I was. Soon enough, neither question was the least bit amusing.

Impotence struck quickly. I checked into the various available remedies, short of a penile implant. These basically consisted of variations on two themes: tourniquets and injections. All were more trouble than they would have been worth even if they had worked, which they didn't. My tremor made injections hopeless. I have about as much chance of successfully injecting a fluid into a sensitive body part as I do of beating Michael Jordan in a slam-dunk contest. Viagra wasn't available when I first needed it, although doctors have since found it quite helpful for their Parkinson's patients. Before Viagra came along, other quick fixes didn't work. The National Parkinson Foundation says there is no evidence that a whole range of putative aphrodisiacs (absinthe, ambergris, animal testes, basil, cannabis, caraway, caviar, clams, coriander, crayfish, cumin, dill, eels, endives, fennel, figs, garlic, ginger, ginseng, juniper, mint, mushrooms, mustard, nutmeg, onions, paprika, prawns, quince, radishes, sesame, shallots, snails, snuff, squid, tarragon, thyme, truffles, and vitamin E) can cut it against Parkinson's disease.[2] The best treatment includes, at the top of the list, frank discussions between sexual partners so that each understands the other's needs. Many experts recommend psychological counseling to address the feelings of depression and inadequacy that are common in Parkinson's and that interfere with sexual relations.[3]

Incontinence arrived more gradually. By now I have the same problem faced by men with prostate cancer: my bladder seems to go from empty to full as fast as a formula-one race car zips from 0 to 60. A warm trickle down the inside of my leg is becoming a familiar sensation, and when I can't get to a bathroom quickly, it can be more than a trickle. Even when I make it to a bathroom on time, there can be more trouble.

If my tremor is active, I face the reverse of the old problem of hitting a moving target from a stationary position: I have to hit a stationary target from a moving position. Sometimes I manage by standing on my left leg, since my right one does most of the shaking. If I don't lose my balance, that works well. If I do, it's a disaster. Increasingly, I must forget my pride and sit on the toilet.

My pride is easier to swallow than my dinner. Parkinson's disrupts the complex series of signals from the brain that tell the throat muscles to contract and push food down the esophagus into the stomach. Food frequently gets stuck halfway down. Sometimes I clear my throat hours after a meal, and some of the last bite suddenly pops up. As a rule, it doesn't taste as good the second time. This problem can become genuinely serious. People with Parkinson's sometimes swallow food down the windpipe instead of the esophagus. If food gets in the lungs, it can trigger an inflammation or become a breeding ground for pneumonia. Speech therapists offer swallowing therapy to teach Parkinson's patients how to avoid this danger. Drooling, particularly during the night, commonly accompanies swallowing problems. If you can't swallow, your saliva collects in your mouth until it overflows. Happily, I have so far dodged this symptom.

My sense of balance is deserting me, particularly when I have progressed from "off" to "on" to hyper. For no apparent reason, I sometimes lurch in one direction or another. Usually I can regain my balance in time to keep from falling over; sometimes, however, I tip over. On one occasion, at a dinner party several years after returning from Brussels, I walked into the dining room from our kitchen, tried to sit down, missed the chair and crashed to the floor. Compounding the danger of a serious fall is low blood pressure, another common side effect. I often feel briefly lightheaded when I get out of bed or rise from a chair, a condition known as orthostatic hypotension. My doctors have warned me that I may black out if I get up too fast. This has happened only once, when a phone call jolted me awake when I was napping on the floor of my Brussels office. I shot up to get the phone and promptly crumpled in a heap back on the floor. Luckily, I woke up again immediately—and meanwhile Isabelle, my office assistant, had answered the phone.

Sleeplessness generally accompanies Parkinson's; it certainly does in my case. In my first year with the disease, one candidate for the office manager's job in Brussels asked me, "How do you sleep if you're always shaking?" I assured her that the minute I lay down, the tremor stopped, allowing me a decent night's sleep. That was true then. Now it's not. Usually I'm so tired when I go to bed that my arms and legs quickly relax. But often they don't stay that way. Typically I get only five or six hours of sleep. When I wake up because I need to go to the bathroom or because my muscles stiffen, I routinely have trouble getting back to sleep. My legs are so shaky that counting backwards by thirteens in French no longer steadies them. But because the Parkinson's tremor is a rest tremor—my arms and legs shake mainly when they're at rest—I can usually control my legs by moving them. Unfortunately, this is no way to sleep. But if I move them for a few minutes—lying on my back and lifting first one knee and then the other—that helps me relax. My right leg is always the last to submit; sometimes, when my left leg has steadied, I conquer my right simply by slightly flexing the muscles that bend it at the knee. With luck, this elaborate strategy delivers another hour or two of sleep—still two or three hours short of what I need. No one in the family ever gets up before me without using an alarm clock.

A lot of research has gone into Parkinson's and sleep. A team of researchers in Norway found that people with Parkinson's were three or four times more likely than other people to suffer from "excessive daytime sleepiness," a scientific phrase that disguises what can be a severe and incapacitating tendency. But surprisingly, Parkinson's patients who slept well at night were just as prone to excessive daytime sleepiness as those who didn't sleep well. Clearly, the cause is something more than sheer exhaustion from a lousy night's sleep, although researchers don't yet know what.[4]

My short intervals of sleep are shortened by an inability to turn while sleeping. Some nights I wake up in exactly the same position in which I went to sleep three or four hours earlier. The extra stiffness makes further sleep more difficult. At least I can turn over when I'm awake. Many people with Parkinson's can't. They need a helping hand or a railing to grab onto simply to get out of bed. As I've said, I also usually wake up more than once to go to the bathroom. Parkinson's advice books recommend urinating completely. They forget that people with Parkinson's don't have good control of the muscles in that part of the body. I find it difficult to get it all out—especially in the middle of the night, when I'm off my medication. As a result, I sometimes find myself waking up hourly and staggering back into the bathroom. The handbooks also recommend keeping a hand-held urine container near the bed so that you don't have to walk to the bathroom so often. I'm afraid that my tremor is so pronounced in the middle of the night that it would render this strategy too risky. But for those whose tremor is not as great as mine, this seems like a good solution.

Still, my sleeping problems remain manageable. Many friends report a fatigue so deep that they can scarcely get up in the morning. That hasn't happened to me. Although I'm drowsy for much of each day, I can generally find enough pep, for example, to play a full round of golf (walking, not riding in a cart) or to put in several consecutive twelve-hour days at work. I simply have to plumb deeper into my energy reserves. Those few researchers who have actually asked Parkinson's patients what bothers them have found low energy at or near the top of most lists. In one study of six Toronto patients whose symptoms ranged from mild tremor to severe disabilities, all six had this complaint. "Normal activities such as eating, dressing, bathing and moving about required enormous amounts of effort."[5] Another group of researchers asked 101 patients to choose any of thirty-nine problems that applied to them. Writing by hand, which was chosen by 93 percent of the patients, topped the list, but "extra physical effort" (82 percent) was second and "lack of energy" (78 percent) was seventh.[6]

Parkinson's also brings weight change—in either direction, but more often down than up. It seems natural that, burning so many calories by shaking, you'd lose weight. That's what has happened to me. Thin as I was before the disease, I've grown thinner still. My family worries that my weight leaves me vulnerable to disease. That's one concern I don't share. Neither do my doctors, who are satisfied that I'm very healthy apart from Parkinson's. Except for contracting tuberculosis in Moscow under taxing conditions, I've barely had so much as a single cold—and never the flu—since the Parkinson's diagnosis. I guess I'm like Judy's mother: while everybody around me gets sick, I'm a poster boy of good health.

I sweat a lot, a common but seldom-discussed Parkinson's symptom, probably because it is so relatively trivial. It's embarrassing—but not much else—to break out in a very visible sweat when you're around strangers. More serious is Parkinson's effect on speech. My voice is often hoarse and low, a condition known as hypophonia. And when I'm trembling, the tremor extends to my talk. Just from hearing me on the phone, some neurologists have guessed that I have Parkinson's.

Only a few of Parkinson's common physical symptoms have failed to find me—and they still have plenty of time to make the scene. The disease robs many people of the full use of their facial muscles, leaving their faces largely without expression. Also damaged is handwriting, which tends to grow progressively smaller (micrographia). But my face is as expressive as it always was (which is to say, not very), and my handwriting, while harder to read than ever, is no smaller than it used to be.

The trouble is that all these symptoms get worse. In my "off" state, my muscle control is diminishing slowly but unmistakably. For the first five years after my diagnosis, I was sufficiently steady in the early morning that I could read and even type. No more: without my pills, I shake too hard to do either. About all I can do at that hour is walk the dog (who, along with the drug companies, is one of the few beneficiaries of my disease).

Parkinson's symptoms are bad enough. But inevitably, the pills we take to control them produce unwelcome side effects. Any time we tinker with one part of the brain, we risk making things worse somewhere else. After the discovery of levodopa, hopes were widespread that this drug would subdue Parkinson's for a lifetime. Those hopes faded quickly. We now know that levodopa gradually causes new problems even as it falters in its principal mission: supplying more dopamine to the brain. After some period—it varies with the individual and can be as long as thirty years—people with Parkinson's have to decide whether levodopa is doing more harm than good.

For most of us, levodopa's first side effects are the involuntary movements known as dyskinesias. Sometimes the whole body writhes and twists from side to side. Sometimes the arms and legs bend in grotesque ways or make sudden, aimless movements. When Michael J. Fox talked about Parkinson's on television in 1999 or 2000, he often bobbed around and couldn't hold still: this too was a form of dyskinesia. Researchers are only now learning how a medication with such promise can cause such grief. The leading theory locates the problem in the brain cells that read the message transmitted by dopamine from the substantia nigra. These cells are accustomed to an even flow of natural dopamine from a healthy substantia nigra. They don't respond well to the on-again, off-again dopamine supply produced by levodopa that is swallowed several times a day.[7]

Levodopa is also disruptive because dopamine serves as a neurotransmitter in other parts of the brain besides the substantia nigra. Researchers have yet to figure out how to deliver levodopa to the area of the brain around the substantia nigra, where dopamine is in short supply, without having it show up elsewhere in the brain, where there is already plenty of dopamine. An excess of dopamine can create, among other things, hallucinations, highly realistic nightmares, delusions, paranoia, and general psychosis.

To make matters worse, levodopa grows less effective at its original mission even as its side effects intensify. Two distinct effects are at work. First, the medication wears off more quickly: where once we could count on three good hours from each pill, we now get two or even less. Second, the medication becomes less predictably effective; I can't count on being as steady five minutes from now as I am now. That's okay as long as I'm writing this book. If I begin shaking in the middle of a paragraph, I can just put the keyboard aside. But it's not okay when I'm driving.

Thirty years after levodopa became available commercially, a lively debate persists over when patients should start taking it. No one knows for sure whether levodopa, which initially improves quality of life in the short term, actually worsens it in the long term by aggravating Parkinson's symptoms and causing nasty side effects. All that's clear is that as time goes by, the ideal range of dopamine in the brain—the amount that produces neither tremor nor dyskinesias—progressively narrows until it is practically impossible to achieve the desired condition. We go straight from underdosed to overdosed; there is no happy medium.

Some experts have argued that levodopa actually kills the nerve cells in the substantia nigra that produce dopamine. The evidence came from laboratory experiments in which rats were fed huge amounts of the drug. More recent studies, however, suggest that levodopa does not kill substantia nigra cells after all.[8] In fact, some experiments on laboratory rats show that levodopa may actually protect the brain cells that manufacture dopamine.[9] Although this argument remains formally unsettled, the weight of the evidence seems to support the view that, at the very least, levodopa does not threaten the neurons in the substantia nigra. Professor David Marsden, my neurologist in London, was a leader among those who support this conclusion.[10]

But there is a more subtle case for delaying levodopa as long as possible. It hinges on the belief, already stated, that levodopa, which clearly improves quality of life in the short term, actually does make it worse in the long term by aggravating Parkinson's symptoms and causing some disabling side effects. Here is the key question: Does levodopa become ineffective and cause dyskinesias and hallucinations after a certain amount of lifetime use? Or is its declining value an inevitable consequence of the disease's progression, unrelated to the amount of past levodopa use? Put differently, would you be just as bad off at this stage if you'd never swallowed a single levodopa pill as if you'd started taking levodopa the moment your Parkinson's was diagnosed?

Intuitively, either explanation for levodopa's declining usefulness makes sense. Many medications—antibiotics, sleeping pills—grow less effective over time; it doesn't seem unreasonable that levodopa would too. On the other hand, it also seems logical that levodopa would lose some of its effectiveness as the disease progresses, regardless of past levodopa use. As more of the substantia nigra's nerve cells die, fewer remain to convert levodopa to dopamine and store the dopamine until the moment it is needed. By this reasoning, levodopa will be less effective five years from now than it is now, regardless of how much of it you take in the meantime.

In the real world, the evidence also seems to point both ways. Several studies suggest that levodopa loses effectiveness and dyskinesias begin when the population of nerve cells in the substantia nigra falls below a threshold.[11] At the same time, recent studies comparing levodopa with the two newest dopamine agonists (pramipexole and ropinirole) found that patients treated with levodopa alone suffered more dyskinesias— and sooner—than those treated with one of the agonists alone. Levodopa, however, also controlled Parkinson's symptoms more effectively. It seems that the price of maximum symptomatic relief is more dyskinesias. But at this early stage of the disease, the dyskinesias are generally not very serious, and it is not clear that those who have them are more likely to develop debilitating dyskinesias later on than those who don't.[12]

Dissatisfied with the general confusion, thirty of the world's leading Parkinson's experts gathered in Paris in January 1998 to try to develop a consensus view that would guide neurologists as they advised their patients. The consensus, if one can be said to have emerged, was that levodopa is not dangerous to Parkinson's patients. But in keeping with the controversy over this question, several of the participants issued minority opinions. Three Americans, for example, wrote, "It has not yet been established that the drug does not have a toxic effect on dopamine neurons." Adding to the doubts, at least in my mind, was the identity of the conference's sponsor: the Swiss drug company Hoffman–La Roche, manufacturer of Sinemet's European equivalent.[13]

Cutting through the fog, University of Maryland neurologist William J. Weiner has written what seems to me to be a sensible summary of the state of knowledge on this crucial issue. Weiner carefully divides the question into two: whether levodopa kills the cells of the substantia nigra, and whether its use accelerates the day when levodopa's side effects will more than offset its ability to mask Parkinson's symptoms. The first question he answers with a resounding no: he finds "no convincing evidence" that levodopa, even in large quantities, has toxic effects on the brains of laboratory animals, much less people. As for the second question, he finds the information generated to date too scant to offer a definitive answer. But this much he can say: early levodopa typically means fewer movement problems but more dyskinesias. Which is the right course for any individual? That depends on individual circumstances.[14]

Unless these questions are authoritatively answered, those of us with the disease are condemned to guessing. Each time we use levodopa, we wonder whether we are advancing the day when the drug will boomerang on us. Each time we forgo another dose, we worry that accepting some discomfort now for some relief later is a delusion. I have followed a common strategy: I take only the minimum of levodopa that I think necessary. Parkinson's or no, I lead a hectic life: working full time, raising three teenagers, and trying to be a decent husband. I can't afford too many underdosed moments. For many years, I got through the early morning hours without any levodopa. While at home, I could shake my way through the morning without too much discomfort or embarrassment, and I could read and get the kids ready for school. Now I can't do either until a half hour after my first levodopa. So I take my first dose immediately after I do my stretching exercises and shave—about ten minutes after I have gotten out of bed. No doubt I would be less shaky if I took some of the stress out of my life. The body responds to stress by releasing extra amounts of certain chemicals—mainly adrenaline but also a number of others including acetylcholine, one of the brain's neurotransmitters. These chemicals put the body on high alert. But they have other effects as well, and one of acetylcholine's is to balance the presence of dopamine in the midbrain. A dopamine shortage upsets that balance and results in the Parkinson's tremor. An extra supply of acetylcholine aggravates the imbalance—and the tremor. That helps explain why I sometimes start to shake the minute I get into a disagreement at work with a reporter who doesn't want to write a story the way I think it should be written. If I avoided this kind of stress, I suppose I'd shake less. But I'd also be more bored and less fulfilled. So far, the extra shakiness is a price I'm willing to pay. There are drugs (Artane and others) to suppress acetylcholine's effect. But they produce grogginess. With anything as complicated as the brain, quick fixes don't exist.

Unfortunately for those who favor dopamine agonists over levodopa, those drugs have some nasty tendencies of their own—although nothing like levodopa's. One group of five researchers reported that nine people taking pramipexole (Mirapex) or ropinirole (Requip), the two newest agonists, suddenly fell asleep at the wheel and crashed.[15] Their vivid language—they described the drivers as targets of "sleep attacks"—caught the attention of the research community. Mere anecdotal evidence, scoffed some. Probably just a case of sleeplessness catching up with a population notorious for sleep deprivation, said others.[16] Maybe so, but a young Maryland doctor with Parkinson's told me he could identify with the targets of sleep attacks. While taking pramipexole, he frequently fell asleep in the middle of the day, particularly when reading. For him, the problem vanished when he switched to ropinirole.

In the end, no medicine has been found that can stop Parkinson's relentless march. After more than a decade, I find its toll increasing on me and everyone around me—mainly my family. Rather than confront stressful situations, I shrink away from them. Pillow talk has almost vanished for Judy and me. By the time I'm in bed, the slightest interruption in my effort to hold still usually activates the tremor. Even before Parkinson's, I was not particularly communicative. Judy must now sometimes think I'm closer to a stone than a husband.

The future no doubt holds more concessions. Nearly everybody I know who was diagnosed before me has ceded more ground. Joan Samuelson, the founder of the Parkinson's Action Network and possibly America's most militant Parkinson's patient, still looks great in her medicated state. But about twelve years from her diagnosis, Joan gave television viewers a glimpse of her condition before her medication kicked in. Sleeping on her stomach, she woke up virtually paralyzed. Only with great effort could she reach the pills that she had left on the nightstand the previous evening. Then she had to lie in bed for forty-five minutes, waiting for the levodopa to find its way to her brain. Only then could she get out of bed.[17] "It's like being a prisoner, and the jail cell is my body," Joan says over the film clip of that scene. Then she talks somberly about her future: "I will slowly slide away. I will lose my capacity to take care of myself, and for some period of time I will disappear, at some point unable to move and speak before I die."

And Joan focused only on physical symptoms. The progression of Parkinson's is sometimes much more than the difference between annoying and crippling physical handicaps. Parkinson's can also ravage the mind. Depression and dementia are its two *D*'s.

Perhaps 40 percent of Parkinson's patients—though estimates run as high as three-quarters—contract depression. Their vulnerability is more than a natural reaction to the knowledge that they have an incurable neurological disease.[18] Parkinson's alters the balance of chemicals throughout the brain, not just in the area that governs movement. One common imbalance is of just the sort that typically causes depression in people without Parkinson's. The good news here is that the same treatments that work for those who don't have Parkinson's should also work for those of us who do. The bad news is that most Parkinson's patients don't seek help for depression, because they regard it as an inevitable reaction to their disease.[19]

Worse than depression is the threat of dementia. What is it? Literally *dementia* means "out of your mind," and Dr. Reich defines it as gradual loss of memory. Dr. Abraham Lieberman, medical director of the National Parkinson Foundation, offers a good description of its practical effects: "Patients may be confused, disoriented, unable to be left alone. They may be agitated, delusional, moody and disinhibited. They usually can't sleep at night and can't stay awake during the day. They may be incontinent of urine and stool." Combining the results of eight studies, Dr. Lieberman estimates that about one-quarter of all Parkinson's patients are demented, the risk increasing with age.[20]

Dana Gunnison worries that today's depression—his most pronounced symptom after three years with Parkinson's—will develop into tomorrow's dementia. Dana, a member of my support group, was diagnosed at 52 in 1997. Some mornings, Dana's depression leaves him unable to muster the energy to go to his job as a social worker for Montgomery County, Maryland. Dana is still not taking levodopa. Physically, he can manage without it. He is right-handed, and so far the disease involves mostly his left side. He also has a boss who promptly said yes when Dana asked for a voice-activated computer. Dana believes that only a finite amount of levodopa will relieve his symptoms over his lifetime. He wants to save it for the day when he needs it to give him the strength to battle dementia. "Like everyone else, I hope for a breakthrough and a cure in my lifetime," he says. "But realistically, I recognize that this probably won't happen. So I want to hold off until I really need it."

Of course, dementia can accompany anyone's old age. To determine Parkinson's impact, researchers at the University of Leeds in England tracked for ten years the experiences of a group of non-demented people with Parkinson's and an otherwise comparable group of non-demented, non-Parkinson's subjects. During the entire period, not one non-Parkinson's subject developed dementia, which the researchers carefully defined according to measures of memory loss and declining intellectual powers. But among the Parkinson's population, more than half had developed symptoms of dementia at the end of the ten years. The most susceptible were older patients with the worst physical disabilities.[21]

Not surprisingly, some of the drugs to control Parkinson's physical disabilities can contribute to our mental disabilities. Artane and the other anticholinergics have been linked to hallucinations, as have selegiline and the dopamine agonists. And levodopa can have disastrous consequences. Dopamine is a vital brain chemical not only in the circuits that control movement but also in those controlling mood and behavior. Levodopa stimulates dopamine production in these circuits as well as in the substantia nigra. Excess dopamine over a long period can produce a wide variety of psychotic behaviors. And short of full-fledged dementia, other mental disabilities threaten. Dr. Lieberman found that more than 20 percent of people with Parkinson's have difficulty organizing their schedule, planning their day, and generally processing information.[22] Whether the cause is the disease or the medication, people forget how to balance a checkbook and do a crossword puzzle, and the quality of their performance at work is likely to decline. This description scares me. I find it increasingly difficult to pack for a vacation or even to remember what to take with me to work in the morning. Judy says this part of my personality is the one that Parkinson's has most changed. My decisiveness, she says, was one of the features that attracted her to me three decades ago: on holiday in Europe, I could drive into a busy, complicated intersection and immediately calculate which way to go. Now I sometimes have a hard time deciding which shirt to wear in the morning.

One bit of good news for me is that my kind of Parkinson's, the kind dominated by the tremor, seems less likely to lead to dementia than does the other variant, whose hallmarks are rigidity, slowness of movement, and depression. The tremor-dominant form of the disease is the more common among those like me who develop Parkinson's at a relatively young age. So, paradoxically, those who contract Parkinson's while they are young are less likely to develop dementia than those who show the symptoms later in life.[23]

And there is good news even for those who do develop dementia as a result of Parkinson's: special medications are available. Traditional drugs to combat dementia prevent dopamine from locking onto the receptor ends of nerve cells all over the brain—not only in the circuits that control mood and behavior but also in those that are responsible for movement. Consequently, they aggravate Parkinson's physical symptoms even as they relieve its mental symptoms. What's needed is a drug that blocks dopamine receptors in the mood and behavior circuits but not in the movement circuits. Several new anti-dementia drugs, notably clozapine (brand name Clozaril), olanzapine (Zyprexa), and quetiapine (Seroquel), are less likely than the traditional drugs to aggravate Parkinson's movement problems. One group of researchers has even reported the case of a patient who drew no benefit from clozapine but considerable relief from quetiapine.[24]

Should people with Parkinson's be told that the disease might one day threaten their mind as well as their body? Don't they have enough to worry about in the present? I remember how determined Dr. Reich was at the time of my diagnosis to discourage me from contemplating a future in a nursing home. He didn't have to lean very hard; I was eager to go into denial. Since then, Dr. Reich has addressed the same subject in a major medical textbook: "With advancing PD (after 10 years), dementia often appears, but it is important to appreciate that *most* patients with PD *do not develop* dementia, and that it is not an inevitable consequence of the disease."[25]

The benefit of not worrying about something you can't do anything about is obvious. But if people with Parkinson's hide their serious symptoms, it is harder to make a case for marshaling the resources to cure their disease. Most of the people with Parkinson's that you see on television don't seem too bad off. Michael J. Fox starred in a television show until he was nine years into the disease, and, as attorney general, Janet Reno held one of the most stressful jobs in the country. If this is the worst the disease can do, many people must wonder, why should medical researchers try very hard to cure it? The answer is that this is not the worst the disease can do, not by a long shot. The Parkinson's Action Network, probably the most effective organization at coaxing more research dollars from Congress, found that it had the most impact when it hit decision-makers over the head with horror stories.[26] It was as a PAN representative that John C. Rogers, a former assistant defense secretary and the son and grandson of people with Parkinson's, testified to a congressional committee: "My father, a World War II veteran, has suffered from Parkinson's for the past 15 years. . . . The 210-pound giant I once knew dropped to 120 pounds before rebounding to a frail 135 pounds. He shakes uncontrollably and suffers from a loss of ambulatory movement, slurred and soft speech, frozen face and freeze-ups. He has experienced severe dementia from his medication and fights depression daily. He has fallen and broken bones just getting out of bed and he has suffered what any one of us would consider egregious indignities to his body. He is also the bravest man I know to have fought this beast every day."[27]

In My Doctors' Words
Dr. Stephen G. Reich, April 22, 1998

For the most part, he is getting along relatively well with no significant change compared to last visit. He finds that he is off first thing in the morning. He has also noticed that he does not feel as sharp in the morning and his best time of day is from 3 to 9 P.M. Emotionally, he is doing well. He is still able to function at an adequate level and his spirits remain up. He finds that he has a fairly smooth response from dose to dose throughout the day with regard to levodopa. His general health has been stable. . . .

In general, Joel looks well and is in good spirits. He is thin but that is his baseline. There is an intermittent rest tremor of the right hand as well as a separate slightly faster bilateral postural and kinetic tremor of the upper limbs. There is mild bradykinesia and cogwheel rigidity. He walks well with no impairment of postural righting reflexes.

Dr. Reich, December 17, 1999

Since his last visit, he is "a little worse." Specifically, he is having predictable off time at end-of-dose [of levodopa], as well as occasional abrupt off periods which are unpredictable but typically follow on the heels of eating more, particularly protein. The off times become so problematic that he has cut back on everything other than local driving and actually took the train here today. When on, he is generally "fine." He does worse in the morning with the shuffling gait, etc. He is still doing fairly well with his activities of daily living, both personally and professionally, but acknowledges being slower. His general health has been stable, and emotionally he continues to do well.

CHAPTER NINE

Keeping the Beast at Bay

Thousands upon thousands of persons have studied disease.
Almost no one has studied health.
— Adelle Davis, *Let's Eat Right to Keep Fit*

EVERY WEEK, EVERY MONTH, EVERY YEAR, the Parkinson's beast grows fiercer. As the symptoms accumulate, adjusting to them becomes progressively more difficult. We become dependent on others to help us do things that healthy adults take for granted—buttoning a shirt, changing a lightbulb, even getting out of bed and feeding ourselves. Our energy deserts us; the smallest chores tire us out. The disease colors the most routine of decisions. Can I safely drive my daughter to her clarinet lesson? Should I have lunch now or wait until after my next dose of levodopa? Insidiously, Parkinson's sometimes takes over the mind along with the body—just when we most need our mental faculties to combat the disease. Depression, dementia, psychosis—how can we manage our physical handicaps if we are burdened by these?

The medical community has understandably spent more time searching for ways to cure us than looking for ways to help us endure the disabilities we have. It has paid scant attention to how people with Parkinson's actually live and how their lives might be improved. The glory is in the curing, not the caring. Jonas Salk is famous for the vaccine that defeated polio, but how many people have ever heard of George Cotzias, whose work with levodopa in the 1960s enables someone like me to work eleven years after my diagnosis? The small academic literature on living with Parkinson's has hardly moved beyond the obvious: that coping grows harder as the disease progresses and that patients become more depressed as their coping mechanisms fail.

At a meeting of my Parkinson's support group, I was astonished to hear a practicing neurologist assail the medical community for these very shortcomings. Dr. Lisa M. Shulman had recently moved (along with Dr. William J. Weiner) from Miami to the University of Maryland, Baltimore; the two of them now run the Movement Disorders Center in Baltimore. "We do a lousy job of providing care for chronic illnesses," she told us. "Our health care delivery system was designed at least a half century ago, when the most pressing health problems were acute illnesses like pneumonia and heart attack, rather than chronic illnesses like Parkinson's disease. Now chronic illnesses represent the great majority of health care needs, but the system continues to care for chronic illness as if it is a series of acute crises. Why? Because that's what the insurance companies will pay for. . . . Instead, we should provide a continuum of care and teach people how to cope and live life well in the face of continuing symptoms." Paradoxically, she said, the groups that strive to cure individual diseases often overlook the more mundane problems of daily living. "There's no reason we can't deal with care and cure at the same time," she said. "It's all very well to work for a cure, but you have to take care of people in the meantime."

The national Parkinson's organizations have tried to fill the void. The American Parkinson Disease Association, for example, has published a series of guides to living with Parkinson's. Some recommendations verge on the absurd: If you're hospitalized and have trouble sleeping, order a backrub, warm milk, or your usual evening cocktail. On holiday, "take along a large mirror to see ceilings of churches while sightseeing."[1] (As Dave Barry would say, I'm not making this up.) Most of the recommendations, however, are sensible: save your high-protein meal for the end of the day so that the protein does not interfere with levodopa; use nonskid rugs, particularly in the bathroom; place nonskid rubber mats on shower and bathtub floors. The APDA handbooks are generally aimed at patients whose symptoms are far more advanced than mine. Thus the ideal bedroom for someone who can't easily roll over or get out of bed includes so many chains and grab bars that it looks a little like an S&M parlor.[2]

The real experts on managing with Parkinson's are the patients themselves—and their spouses and other caregivers. If there are a million Americans with Parkinson's, there are a million styles of dealing with the disease. No two Parkinson's patients have exactly the same symptoms; no two have the same personal resources to summon. Yet in my experience, those who seem to lead the most fulfilling lives have several characteristics in common.

For one, they stay active. It doesn't so much matter what they do as that they do something. Some are still on the job twenty years after the first symptoms of their disease. Others quit working and take up poetry or even (now here's a challenge for a trembling hand) painting. If they don't get enough exercise in the ordinary course of the day, they force themselves to do whatever they are capable of doing, whether that means swimming laps or just sitting still and turning their head from side to side.[3]

It's so tempting for people with Parkinson's just to curl up at home rather than summon the extra energy to do something new—especially because energy is one of the disease's first casualties. Dr. Lucien Cote, a New York City neurologist, has found that many Parkinson's patients avoid the unfamiliar: "They experience apprehension at undertaking just about anything." Ironically, he says, Parkinson's is actually more disruptive when we are at home than when we go out, because it particularly affects the brain circuitry responsible for the subconscious movements that we use in the familiar terrain of our homes. "I am constantly convincing PD patients and their families not to give up a planned journey and, once they have taken the trip, they are usually pleased to have done it," Cote says.[4]

Those who have the most success at coping with Parkinson's tend to be the ones with deep reservoirs of religious faith. A sense of perspective also helps. Those who don't take themselves too seriously seem better off than those who ponder why the disease struck them and not someone else. Parkinson's changes your life, but it doesn't destroy the opportunity for accomplishment, contribution, pleasure, and love. A related asset is a sense of humor. Morris Udall, who served in Congress for about twelve years after developing Parkinson's, was there when some of his colleagues were found to be having affairs with a particularly well-proportioned lobbyist named Paula Parkinson. He said he knew about two kinds of Parkinson, and both left him shaky.

Some external factors also play a role. A supporting family goes a long way toward making life with Parkinson's livable. And a sense of financial security helps a great deal: not only is Parkinson's expensive to treat, but it also sharply reduces the earning potential of those who have it. I've had the good fortune to encounter many inspiring individuals who have refused to let Parkinson's get the better of them. One of my favorites is Tom Collins, a fellow patient of Dr. Reich at Johns Hopkins.

There is nothing superhuman about Tom Collins. I met him on the front porch of his modest wood-frame house along a busy road midway between Washington and Baltimore—a house close enough to the highway that a car once crashed through the living room. He showed the signs of a long relationship with levodopa: the same sort of writhing, twisting motions with his limbs and torso that afflict me when my levodopa level is too high. The son of a West Virginia coal miner, Tom married shortly after high school, moved to the Baltimore-Washington area, and became first a schoolteacher and then a salesman. At his peak, he supervised 169 sellers of cleaning and janitorial supplies. Then, in 1984, he noticed slight twitches in his right hand and foot. At age 50, his condition was diagnosed as Parkinson's.

His first instinct, typical of the newly diagnosed, was to check the literature. His reaction was also standard: "It scared the bejeezus out of me." The same thing would later happen to me, and I would flee to Brussels to forget the disease. Collins confronted it directly and, finding no local Parkinson's support groups in his area, promptly organized one. "Somebody once told me, 'You're the only fellow I know who'd go out and catch a disease and make a project out of it,' " he chuckled. "But I find it therapeutic. It doesn't leave me time to sit around and do nothing. If you quit and give up, it'll get you. . . . I'd take a break, but I'm scared to."

Tom receives Social Security disability benefits and income from an annuity he bought before he developed Parkinson's. His wife, Sue, who was successfully treated for breast cancer in 1991, is the chief election clerk in Maryland's Howard County. Her job pays well and provides the insurance that covers Tom's medications, which he figures cost $11,000 a year. What sacrifices has Tom made to his disease? Precious few. "I don't change lightbulbs," he said. "But I haven't given up anything really important." A heavy-set man, he still swims, lifts weights, and plays golf—although usually just ten or twelve holes instead of eighteen.

All these activities require more effort than they used to. "The little things you take for granted become real chores, like washing a car. And it took me a whole day to paint this porch instead of the hour it would have taken. It's like you're always bucking a strong headwind, always pushing uphill. But there's no going back. You've got to be proud of what you can do today and not measure it against what you used to be able to do. I don't think I'm doing too bad for sixteen years with the disease. A lot of it is staying active. When you're busy helping other people, you don't have time to feel sorry for yourself."

Tom and Sue, whose two grown sons live nearby, regularly attend their Methodist church. "You have to have faith in something more than yourself," Tom said. "I have to admit I sometimes asked myself, 'Why me?' I'd buy a plug of tobacco and sit on a stump and wonder about that. Then I realized Sue and I could be a lot worse off. The Lord hasn't let us down yet."

Rusty Glazer, like Collins, participates in support groups but, unlike Collins, is one of those exceptional people with Parkinson's who seem to have controlled their disease completely. I've rarely seen him display any symptoms. Although he's my age and has had the disease as long, he manages on half as much medicine. He attends support group meetings not so much to find help as to offer it. A frequent public speaker, he stresses the value of a positive outlook, a sense of humor, and personal dignity. Only when I knew him well did I realize the difficulty he had experienced to achieve his present calm.

Rusty was 47 in 1991 when he got his diagnosis: the mysterious movement difficulties on his left side and his feeling of being continually washed out were the result of more than a stressful life. His reaction was the opposite of mine. Instead of sharing the news with friends, relatives, and colleagues at Congress's General Accounting Office, he guarded it closely. "I was ashamed of the fact that I had an illness for which there was no known cure," he told me much later. "I became obsessed with my appearance and how others, especially my colleagues at work and at temple, might respond to me." For someone serving as president of a 1,500-member professional organization and as a board member of his synagogue, he found it difficult to maintain appearances. And at home, his wife and teenage daughter provided him not with emotional support but with criticism that he was living like a hermit.

Rusty went public only after two of his friends died, one of AIDS and the other—Sid Dorros, his mentor and sole confidant—of septic shock brought on by Parkinson's-induced constipation. Chosen to deliver the eulogy at Dorros's funeral, Rusty committed himself to work for a cure. He promptly became a highly visible figure in Parkinson's circles. Previously he shunned support groups: "I didn't want to be around a lot of sick people." Now he organized one in northern Virginia for young people and served as president of the local chapter of the American Parkinson Disease Association. His profile was so high that a friend once described him as a "Parkinson's disease groupie."

Like most Parkinson's patients I've met who seem to have asserted full control over their lives, Rusty professes strong religious faith. "I don't see how people get along without it," he said. "You have to believe in a Supreme Being, someone you can turn to and pray to. . . . I'm God's child." Why did God let him get this terrible disease? Asking why God does anything is a waste of time, he said. We may never know God's reasons. "I keep busy simply fighting the inclination to let the illness absorb me. I'd much rather use the time the good Lord has given me to be as productive as I can, have fun in the process, and not worry about the future."

A surprising number of those who have aggressively gone public about their Parkinson's were once, like Rusty, intensely private. The most famous example is actor Michael J. Fox. Fox, who was just 30 years old when diagnosed with Parkinson's in 1991 (and who still looks barely old enough to vote), stayed silent for more than seven years before publicly revealing his condition in 1998. When he established the Michael J. Fox Foundation for Parkinson's Research in 2000, he immediately became the world's most prominent anti-Parkinson's crusader.

Pittsburgh's Jim Cordy, a former metallurgist who got his diagnosis at the age of 40, is another. Having seen him repeatedly lobby Congress for more Parkinson's research money, I had assumed that Jim had always been public about his disease. Not so. He spent seven years keeping it a secret. His Parkinson's was diagnosed one week after returning from his honeymoon with his second wife. His principal symptoms were fatigue ("the feeling you get after Thanksgiving dinner, times ten") and a lack of facial expression, but neither made his ailment obvious. So he kept working for steelmaker Allegheny Ludlum, binding to silence the only colleague he informed. Finally, the Parkinson's became overwhelming. He had to retire on his disability insurance, which replaced two-thirds of his salary. Leaving the pressure cooker of the office, he said, immediately alleviated his symptoms: "There's no way of appreciating what that stress does to you until you get out from under it."

Deciding to build a Japanese garden in his yard, he discovered, over the garden fence, that two of his neighbors were neuroscientists at the University of Pittsburgh. They introduced him to Michael Zigman, Pitt's chief Parkinson's researcher. Together, Cordy and Zigman decided to raise money for a chapter of the American Parkinson Disease Association. From that start, Jim became an activist. He testifies before Congress and lobbies for more research funds. When Parkinson's patients wanted a new organization—one not dominated by doctors—Jim was a founding member. In effect, he's devoted his life to help find a cure. "I figure anything I do is something that otherwise wouldn't have been done. What I don't do wouldn't have been done anyway, so I don't worry about it."

Of course, not all Parkinson's patients initially hide their disease. Perry Cohen, the leader of my support group, became outspoken almost immediately after his diagnosis in 1996. I'm pleased to have played a small role in his decision. A mutual friend steered Perry to me for advice, and I suggested that he sign up with the Parkinson's Action Network, the most militant Parkinson's organization. Several other people gave him similar advice. He attended PAN's 1996 "public policy forum," where participants learned congressional lobbying techniques. The first person Perry met was Jim Cordy, who had been an undergraduate a year behind Perry at Carnegie-Mellon University. Perry slipped easily into the new group.

With a Ph.D. in organizational studies from the Massachusetts Institute of Technology, Perry had grown weary of his consulting business, which evaluated management structures in government agencies. Disability insurance and a working wife meant he could work almost full-time on the Parkinson's crusade. Finding no support group in Washington for people, like us, afflicted early in life, he started the group that now includes me. He joined the lobbying campaign for the Udall bill (named for Morris K. Udall) authorizing $100 million specifically for Parkinson's research. A native of Atlanta, he helped get the Parkinson's lobby to see then-House Speaker Newt Gingrich, who comes from the Atlanta suburbs. And Congress did enact the Udall bill.

Perry regards lobbying the way I regard writing this book: a means of resisting his condition without being immobilized by it. "In an odd way, my lobbying is a way to avoid thinking about my problem," he said. "And it was something I could do that would affect my future. . . . I was in the right place at the right time."

To me, the most fascinating celebrity coping story is that of the former attorney general Janet Reno. Where most Parkinson's patients are embarrassed by their tremor, she seems oblivious. Where most people avoid stress, as attorney general she rushed from one controversy to another—from the firebombing of the Branch Davidian compound to the custody battle over little Elian Gonzalez. Where most people keep a low public profile, she was all over the 6 o'clock news. I was the first writer to interview her about Parkinson's, and I found her story no less extraordinary than the image of this imposing woman on my TV screen.

Typically, her first symptom was trivial: in March of 1995, her left forefinger and thumb began tapping together involuntarily. By October, the trembling in her left hand was bad enough to send her to her doctor, who referred her to a neurologist. The neurologist immediately diagnosed Parkinson's and prescribed a low dose of levodopa. Expecting to spend her life in Miami after her stint as attorney general, she switched to a Miami neurologist, who stopped the levodopa and prescribed first selegiline and then Mirapex. During the Elian Gonzalez affair she took no levodopa at all! Only in mid-2000 did she begin taking two levodopa pills of 100 milligrams each to supplement the Mirapex. Such a low dose works because she is remarkably unselfconscious about her tremor. "It doesn't bother me," she said. "I've been walking through airports and seen myself on TV monitors and been surprised at how visible the tremor was."

Essentially, she disdains medication. "I learned long ago to take a deep breath, wiggle, relax, and do the best I can." (By wiggle she means letting her hands dangle at her sides and wiggling them.) She has made almost no concessions to the disease. "I still climb mountains," she said. She began kayaking at about the time she was diagnosed; she hasn't given that up either. "I'm not as graceful as I used to be," she said, "but I was never very graceful." In one very small respect the disease has taken a toll. "I can ride a horse very well, but now I can no longer lift my leg over the horse. Recently I went to the [U.S.-Mexican] border to thank the Border Patrol for their services. I wanted to ride a horse along the border, but I couldn't get my leg over the horse's back. So I stood on a chair and was able to get on just fine."

When Reno received her diagnosis, she immediately told her family and close co-workers, including President Clinton, whom she described as highly supportive. She recalled that Sen. Alan Simpson, a now-retired Wyoming Republican, called her on the day her diagnosis became public. Someone had told him he should pray for her. "Prayer, hell, she doesn't need our prayers," she quoted Simpson as saying. "My father was a United States senator with Parkinson's, and it never bothered him. When he shook, all he did was say he had a phantom wing." Still, Reno went to the bookshelves to see what the disease might have in store for her, and her first reaction was "Yeoww!" But her neurologist thought her kind of Parkinson's would progress slowly, and he predicted that she wouldn't be seriously disabled for twenty years. With that prognosis, she doesn't feel very sorry for herself. "I think of all the things that beset people," she said. "We all die of something."

I told her that parts of the Parkinson's community had criticized her for not becoming, like Michael J. Fox, a forceful advocate for more money to fight the disease. "There will be an appropriate time for that," she replied, "but right now my duty is to all the American people, and I can't engage in activity on behalf of only some of them." She said she thought she served a larger purpose by being a role model, demonstrating that people with Parkinson's can still live life to the fullest.

Even after leaving office as attorney general, Reno showed no sign that her disease had got the better of her. Far from retreating from the public eye, she ran for governor of Florida—an exhausting, stressful pursuit if ever there was one. Ron Brownstein, the political reporter in the *Los Angeles Times* Washington bureau, described her as being as steady as a rock in a strong current. "If it weren't for the tremor," he told me in the office one day, "she wouldn't move at all."

I don't mean to leave the impression that everyone who struggles against Parkinson's prevails. One young woman who seemed to have triumphed was Paige Bremer of Scottsdale, Arizona, diagnosed at 24. To those who knew her, she was "exuberant" and "vivacious," adjectives that would apply to few with the disease. At 31, she was planning to be married, in late 2000. For her "bachelorette" party, she planned to hike into the Grand Canyon. She ran her own Internet site—an electronic support group that she called The Park Place. "I am here to tell you that having a chronic illness is not the end of the world, but an incredible learning experience," she wrote on her website. She described her operation (deep brain stimulation) in 1999 to relieve the tremor: how she and her family had joked about it as the operation approached, how much better it made her feel. After the operation, she wrote, "as they wheeled me to the Intensive Care Unit (ICU), I saw my family and friends with smiles on their faces. I smiled right back at them and said, 'Hi! That was fun! I'm hungry!'" Then one day in June of 2000, on the eve of a trip to Washington for the Parkinson's Action Network's annual lobbying blitz, Paige left her clothes neatly folded on her bed, went into her garage, closed the door, turned on the car, and died of carbon monoxide poisoning.

What a horrible demonstration of the terror that lurks just below the surface in all of us! Paige seemed to have everything going for her: a loving family, an active life, a sense of humor, a determination not to take herself too seriously. She seemed to have done everything right. But those who knew her said depression, which so often accompanies Parkinson's, began sinking its hooks into Paige a year and a half before her death. Her open defiance of the disease, which until then had accurately reflected her state of mind, became a mask to hide her distress. "Her exuberance was a smokescreen," said Barbara Gormly, a Parkinson's patient who was Paige's mentor. "It was as if she was playing a role in the theater," said Stephanie Fromer, a Californian who was to be Paige's hotel roommate in Washington for the PAN action. "Finally she just couldn't keep it up any more."

Her fiancé, Paul Ketchum, said Paige's story was more complicated. She had a rocky childhood, Paul said, and as an adult she had become a compulsive gambler. At the gaming tables, she found she could concentrate so hard that she could forget, ever so briefly, her illness. But she had also run up serious debts, a factor that Paul said was weighing on her mind when she walked into the garage that June day. "She was a wonderful girl who got very confused and very depressed," Paul said. "Everybody around her loved her, but she didn't love herself."

Many Parkinson's patients go outside traditional medicine, often in desperation, to find ways to improve their condition. My neurologist, Dr. Reich, directed a study that found that 40 percent of a sample of patients resorted to herbal medicine, vitamins, massage, acupuncture, or some other form of alternative therapy—and half the patients didn't tell their neurologists. On average, people who experimented were more educated and wealthier than those who did not. They had also developed the disease at a relatively young age.[5]

Dr. Reich's collaborator, a medical student named Pam Rajendran, found one 45-year-old man who had tried fourteen forms of alternative therapy, from vitamins to acupuncture. A man in his 50s had developed a unique regimen to combat stress: two hours of video games early in the morning and two hours more before bed. She also found people who were eager to cash in on other people's desperation. Visiting an alternative medicine store, she asked a salesman to recommend products that would help with Parkinson's disease. He recommended no fewer than thirteen, from milk thistle to ginkgo biloba, at a monthly cost of $263.29. I have found no convincing scientific evidence that any of these treatments does any good. But clearly, with Americans pouring $27 billion a year into alternative medicine for all types of disorders, many people think it helps them individually. One of the regulars in my support group swears by acupuncture, and her experience prompted me to try it and see what would happen.

There's no mistaking Dr. Jing N. Wu's office for Dr. DC's. Dr. Wu works out of a house in residential Washington. Past the reception area and the waiting room, I am shown to a treatment room furnished with only the basics: a wooden desk, a folding chair for the doctor, a second chair for the patient, and a rollaway bed with a stool at its foot. The walls are not cluttered with diplomas and other certificates; the only decoration is a pair of framed watercolors of ducks. Blinds, not curtains, cover the only window. The other lighting comes from a ceiling fixture; only one of its two bulbs is working.

Dr. Wu strides briskly into the room, says a quick hello, and gets down to business. He is a formidable figure: nearly six feet tall and large-boned. His voice is rich but gentle; his English, without accent. He takes my pulse in both wrists and then asks if I've had any eye problems recently. Impressed, I respond that I've had cataracts removed from both eyes in the past year. He's not surprised. "There are twelve pulses," he says mysteriously, "and the one that includes your eyes is aberrant." Then he has me slip off my shoes and socks, roll up my sleeves, and lie on the bed. As he inserts thirteen needles—from four in my feet to one on top of my head—he explains: "Unlike Western medicine, which treats disease, Chinese medicine treats the whole body. We try to strengthen the body so that the body is able to conquer the disease."

I lie on the bed for about fifteen minutes until Dr. Wu returns. Removing all the needles except the one on top of my head, he says he wanted the needles to be in place for half of a twenty-eight-minute body cycle. Then he inserts three needles into the back of my neck and, after no more than a minute or two, removes them and the one on top of my head.

"We changed your body energy down to theta," he says. His first goal, he says, will be to enable me to get enough sleep. (A recent study of twenty Parkinson's patients treated by acupuncture found that sleep improved but all of their Parkinson's movement disorders were no better after the treatment than before.)[6] He informs me that Western societies have established a daily routine that works against the body's natural rhythms, which include an after-lunch siesta that has been programmed into our genes to renew our energy levels. "But Henry Ford changed all that, and now we treat our bodies as if they were machines coming off an assembly line that we can run any way we want."

When I return for my second session two weeks later, I feel essentially unchanged from before my first. Certainly I have slept no better. Dr. Wu again takes my pulses. Then, after I stretch out on the bed, he uses more needles—probably fifteen to twenty; I can't keep count—and seems to put more on the right side (the shaky side) than the left. This time, some go in my legs. And he leaves them in for more than twenty-eight minutes, long enough for me to get a good nap.

As he takes the needles out, he explains that my pulse showed a different field of distress this time: the stomach field as opposed to the gallbladder field. Both run from head to foot, but by different routes. These fields are like channels along which energy circulates. There are twelve such fields on each side of the body, he says, and they correspond to the twelve pulses. Two others run up the center of the body, one up the front and one up the back. Altogether, these fourteen fields have 411 node points, or energy points, and it is here that the needles are inserted.

"Chinese medicine treats process rather than system," he says. "We don't treat a heart attack just by treating the heart; we treat the entire energy field that includes the heart." He adds that he is now studying "visualization" as a means by which one can make oneself healthier. The practitioner, he says, must "visualize" the part of the body that is not performing properly and, by sheer willpower, force it to do its job better. On one recent night he was reading an English-language version of a text on visualization when he heard a voice say, "They have translated me badly." So he went to the original Chinese and found, sure enough, that the translation was sloppy. Now he's working on a better one.

For my third session Dr. Wu seems in a hurry and, after taking my twelve pulses, ducks my questions about what they reveal. The needles this time total sixteen, including one on top of my head and one in the middle of my forehead. He leaves them in for a good ten minutes more than twenty-eight minutes before asking me to be careful to note any changes in my condition over the next seventy-two hours.

No changes develop. I'm not entirely surprised. Before seeing Dr. Wu I had vowed to treat acupuncture seriously. It's easy for science-steeped Westerners to make fun of it. But if there were nothing to it, why did James Reston, the late *New York Times* columnist and Washington bureau chief, find that acupuncture alleviated his pain after an emergency appendectomy while he was covering one of President Nixon's early trips to China in 1971? Why would so many people I know and respect say it has helped them manage their Parkinson's? Why would my health insurance company, which is always reaching for reasons not to pay, cover twenty visits a year to an acupuncturist? I didn't want to deny acupuncture a chance to work for me.

At the same time, I wanted some kind of Western explanation of cause and effect: why should a fistful of needles stuck in my body in the morning help me sleep better at night? I concluded that no such explanation exists: you accept acupuncture on its own terms or not at all. For me, its own terms are decidedly bizarre: about bodily channels of energy, many of them extending from head to toe; about "acupoints" along these channels, where acupuncture needles can facilitate healing; about the balance between "yin" and "yang," where yin is female and dark and winter, and yang is male and light and summer. None of this is measurable, at least not by the West's scientific instruments. Why does acupuncture work? Even its advocates can't explain it. "The understanding of how acupuncture works is in the very earliest stages of development and requires more resources and talent if it is to be explored properly," write the authors of the latest acupuncture text to be found at the National Library of Medicine. "Regardless of the current state, negative conclusions are unjustified. Put in the vernacular, there is too much smoke to discount fire."[7]

In my case, there isn't much fire. On my fourth visit, Dr. Wu determines from my pulses that my kidney and bladder channels (both in the yang category) are overactive and my liver channel (a yin) is underactive. But my tremor, less than fully controlled by my medications, defies his attempts to place needles in the appropriate points on my feet and legs. He tries to compensate with two needles in the top of my head. But to no avail: only when my standard medicine finally goes to work am I steady enough for the needles. My encounter with acupuncture ends with Dr. Wu removing the needles and sending me home.

We patients are by no means the only ones who have to learn to cope with a degenerative disease. In some ways, family members—particularly spouses and children—have a harder role. Within weeks of my diagnosis, Judy and I attended simultaneous Parkinson's seminars, one for patients and the other for their spouses, at Johns Hopkins. I emerged from mine feeling moderately upbeat; those who had had the disease a lot longer than I appeared to be functioning all right, and they had some sensible ideas about how to manage their lives. Judy, by contrast, looked awful. She had been subjected to hours of complaining by people who felt their lives closing in around them as they spent more and more of their time tending to their spouse. At that moment I vowed not to turn her into my nursemaid. So far, I think I've succeeded pretty well. I can't drive long distances by myself, but it's my daughter Anne as often as Judy who goes with me. And I've shed the annual burden of preparing our tax returns, but that's fallen to an accountant. I believe I've continued to do my share of the housework.

My disease still has a long way to go, however, and the real test will come only when I'm considerably more disabled than now. There's no predicting what awaits her. Caregivers are the forgotten victims of Parkinson's and all other chronic diseases, the persons who are expected to suffer in saintly silence as they devote twenty-four hours a day to their ill relatives. Chris McGonigle, who endured fifteen years of hell between her husband's diagnosis of multiple sclerosis at age 32 and his death, looked everywhere for advice on how to cope with someone whose illness had made him violent and dangerous. All she found were "impossibly cheery" books full of tips on how to care for a loved one: nothing on raising your children, managing your finances, coping with your anger, or pursuing your sex life. So she wrote a book herself, to dispel the myth that caregiving provides satisfaction enough. "The notion that we might aspire to lives beyond that of fulltime caregivers doesn't seem to occur to professionals," McGonigle wrote.[8] In her lone example involving Parkinson's, a young husband becomes violent and psychotic before the long-suffering wife finally realizes there is nothing she can do for him and commits him to a nursing home.

Fortunately, most Parkinson's family stories are not so dramatic. Even so, the ordinary caregiving life can be arduous. In a study of German caregivers from both inside and outside the family, more than 70 percent of all the caregivers reported psychological stress—and 94 percent of those who were caring for someone with depression or dementia. Anxiety feeds anxiety in a vicious circle: distressed patients upset and disorient their caregivers, whose increasing isolation, anger, and sense of inadequacy exact a further toll on the patients.[9]

Just as Parkinson's patients are the leading experts on coping with the disease, their spouses and children know more than anyone else about caring for them. That means three of the nation's top experts live right here in the Washington area. Morton Kondracke, a leading Washington journalist (and briefly a colleague of mine when we both worked for the Chicago Sun-Times in the late 1960s), is the author of *Saving Milly: Love, Politics, and Parkinson's Disease*, a moving story of Mort's love for his Parkinson's-afflicted wife and his effort to get more governmental financial support for the battle against the disease.[10] Susan Hamburger, the wife of Stan Hamburger, a twenty-year patient, writes a monthly column on caregiving for the National Parkinson Foundation website.[11] And Donna Dorros, widow of Sid Dorros, whose inspirational book on combating Parkinson's was one of the first to be written from a patient's point of view,[12] still runs a support group every Wednesday morning that she and her husband started in 1985. She invites caregivers as well as patients.

The first time I attended Donna's group, I naturally wondered why she was still devoting so much time to people with whom she had no direct connection since her husband's death. "It has given me a real sense of purpose in my life," she explained. "I have a storehouse of knowledge and experience that I think would be criminal not to share." Most of the support group's members were older than 60, and their Parkinson's was more advanced than mine. Each was asked to talk about something that had happened during the week since the last meeting.

Polly, a small, serious-looking woman, described her hallucinations, which have plagued her for some years. "A family sits in my living room," she said. "It's a large family, with a lot of children who aren't very well behaved. They come at 7 or 8 in the morning and stay until midnight, mostly parked in front of the television."

Tom, his head hanging down, said nothing. His wife, Annabelle, spoke for the family. The issue for her was the absence of places—and staff members familiar with Parkinson's—to which she could entrust Tom's care for anywhere from a few hours to a few weeks. Sometimes she needed to lead a life of her own. In the past, she said, a family member or friend would stay with Tom so that she could run errands, go to a movie, or even take a short vacation. Now she was planning a two-week vacation and, for the first time, would leave Tom in an assisted-living facility. She worried that Tom wouldn't like it, but she was desperate for a break from the numbing routine of caregiving.

Years of experience have taught Annabelle another lesson of caregiving: don't overdo it, not only for your own sake but for the patient's. People with Parkinson's need to feel some sense of independence, no matter how small. "Tom used to spend half an hour buttoning his shirt," she said. "At first I tried to help him, but I've learned that he needs to do it for himself if he can." At that point Donna said, "I never did anything for Sid without asking first."

In his book, Sid tells a harrowing story about the wives of two of his roommates at the hospital where all three had had operations to relieve their Parkinson's tremors in 1967. One blamed her husband for faking his symptoms to spite her; the other blamed her mother-in-law for somehow inducing her husband's illness. Sid wondered if the burden of caring for their husbands had so strained these two women that they cracked.

Someone who has kept her composure is Susan Hamburger, whose website column about caregiving is a nice mix of personal experience and practical tips. Susan, who turned 60 in 1999, figures her childhood perfectly equipped her to be a caregiver. "I had a difficult mother," she explained. Her mother suffered from depression and made it a practice to compete with Susan, the only girl among her three children. Part of the competition involved a steady stream of criticism of her daughter. "If I could cope with her," Susan said, "I can manage just about anything."

For years there was no need to. She and Stan were living in the Washington area in 1980 while Stan, then a periodontist, commuted to Baltimore's Johns Hopkins University to study epidemiology. Going back to school was hard for a 45-year-old, and the commute wasn't easy. When Stan became exhausted and depressed, his doctor blamed stress. But Susan and Stan, unconvinced, consulted a neurologist, who quickly diagnosed Parkinson's. Their first coping strategy resembled mine: they went about their business and saved the worrying for later. "Was I in denial? Maybe, but I'm not sure," Susan wrote in her first column. "Maybe denial is okay if it helps us deal with something that is psychologically overwhelming and allows us to absorb the new reality a little at a time."

Despite his Parkinson's, Stan became an epidemiologist, and Susan, then an elementary school psychologist, switched careers and became a statistician for the National Institutes of Health. In 1991, as Stan's condition deteriorated, she happened to read about Joan Samuelson's efforts to get more money from Congress for Parkinson's—and contacted her. Susan was one of a few dozen persons who attended Joan's first annual "public policy forum." Participants learned about lobbying techniques and the current state of Parkinson's research, before descending on members of Congress to make their case. "Becoming active wasn't anything I intended to do," Susan said. "I didn't even think of myself as a caregiver until the last couple of years."

She does now. Stan has great difficulty walking and frequently needs a wheelchair, and his short-term memory has virtually disappeared. But the two of them still go almost everywhere together. I see them mostly at Parkinson's-related events, but when Susan goes to the grocery store or the doctor's office, Stan is generally with her. Her caregiving philosophy rests on the simple conviction that the recipient must have confidence in the love and devotion of the giver. "The one important message that I wanted Stan to really understand from the very beginning was that I loved him and would always be there for him . . . ," she wrote. "I knew that if I had a serious illness, I would be comforted by hearing this, so I talked to him daily about how we were going to deal with each change as it happened and that we were going to do it together."

Judy has not made a point of talking with me every day about how we're in this together. She doesn't have to. I know it implicitly. Without her, I'm not sure what kind of a mess I'd be today. It wouldn't be pretty.

In My Doctors' Words
Dr. Stephen G. Reich, June 6, 2001

Although in general he is still getting along relatively well, both personally and professionally, there are some specific problems he brings up today. First thing in the morning is a difficult time with regard to shaving, and he is a bit more concerned about his safety in the shower. He has no difficulty initiating sleep, but generally wakes up within four hours for unclear reasons, and often, but not always, has trouble getting back to sleep. The main culprit seems to be that during these times, he starts to worry about things and will often get out of bed and engage. Yet, part of the problem seems to relate to Parkinson's itself, making it difficult to shift positions in bed. . . .

There is occasional end-of-dose wearing off [of levodopa], but in general, he is off for no more than one hour total per day except during very stressful days, when it may be as much as three to four hours. He finds that walking helps when the tremor is severe. Since last visit, Joel tried stopping the Artane, which worsened the tremor. He has had no falls. He is still independent with his personal and professional activities of daily living. He still is very conscientious about following a protein redistribution diet. His general and emotional health have been stable. . . .

Joel fluctuated while here today, initially having a severe tremor, which gradually resolved. There is little, if any, bradykinesia. Toward the end of the examination, he began to develop mild dyskinesias but was able to walk well, without any impairment of balance.

Joel is now 12 years into Parkinson's disease and is still functioning at a fairly good level.

CHAPTER TEN

Tomorrow's Remedies

To extreme diseases, extreme and exquisite remedies are best.
—Hippocrates, Greek physician

IN MY NAÏVE EARLY YEARS with Parkinson's disease, when people asked how I could live with the knowledge that, probably for the rest of my life, I would always be sicker next week than this, I had a ready answer. "Right now I can manage just fine with the drugs available today," I'd say. "And by the time those drugs can no longer do the job, I'm counting on medical science to have come up with something better."

For some years, this comforting notion allowed me to cruise along without too much worrying. I could follow my star to Brussels while the medical research community crafted a cure. In Brussels I went about my exhilarating business without letting Parkinson's possess me. Back in Washington, I relied on the treatments that were available when I was diagnosed. I was nearly ten years into the disease before I began taking tolcapone, the first medicine unlike anything available in 1990. But now, eleven years from my diagnosis as I write this, my day of reckoning may be approaching. Medical science doesn't have much time if it is to rescue me from Parkinson's worst ravages.

Perhaps I will be blessed. The doggedness of Parkinson's advocates has loosed an avalanche of research money. In 1998, Congress dramatically increased the budget of the National Institutes of Health for combating Parkinson's.[1] Along with the money, a sense of euphoria washed over the Parkinson's community. Compared with the past, the research resources seemed so vast that they inspired predictions of victory early in the new century. Dr. Gerald Fishbach, then the director of NIH's center for neurological disorders, was asked at a Senate hearing in September 1999 how long it might take to "conquer" Parkinson's. "I think with all the intensive effort, with a little bit of skill and luck, five to ten years is not unrealistic," he said. "We will do everything possible to reduce that below five years. I wouldn't rule that out."

I hope he's right. As I write in 2001, there is still no reliable way to stop or even slow Parkinson's relentless progression, much less reverse it. After so many years of watching promised cures come to nothing, I've begun to wonder. I'm not even sure what *cure* means any more. Arresting the disease's progress? Reversing the symptoms? Eliminating them? You can cure an infectious disease such as tuberculosis by taking enough antibiotics to destroy the infection. Broken bones heal, and you can have surgery to remove cataracts that once blinded and to repair broken hips that crippled. But with Parkinson's, there is no foreign agent to kill, no bone to heal. There are only knots of dead or dying brain cells. Restoring the brain to its pre-Parkinson's condition would involve replacing or reviving huge numbers of dead or dying cells. If medical science achieves that, I don't expect it in my lifetime. Less ambitious goals include retarding the disease's progress (symptoms would mount, but more slowly), halting its progress (symptoms would be frozen), and reversing some of the disease's damage (symptoms would improve). For myself, I'd settle for anything that merely stopped the disease's progress; I can live pretty well the way I am. But this is too little for the many whose Parkinson's is more advanced. They need to turn the clock back to a time when they remained at least minimally independent. And they need to do it quickly, lest the disease outrun the remedy.

I have plenty of company in my sense that time is running short. Ed Calhoon, who is my age and whose diagnosis followed mine by two years, has also watched promised cures come and go. He committed his feelings to verse:

> Trials of new meds
> most with no free lunch
> but new side effects
> to offset the gains.
> Promises of a cure,
> and research saying
> that genes play a part,
> only leading to the
> fear I may have passed on
> the disease to my daughter,
> in addition to bipolar disease
> she already got
> like her cousin.
> Support groups,
> where many are

worse off than me,
and surgery or meds
that work for one person
don't work for another.
Claims that longevity
is not affected by the disease,
followed by obituaries
that state the deceased
had the disease,
but died of something else.
(coincidence? I think not.)
Pray and pay for the cure.

How often have potential new treatments seemed just around the corner, only to recede mysteriously? When I got my diagnosis in 1990, a new medication called selegiline was thought to slow the disease's progression. Now that notion has been widely discredited. In 1996, when researchers announced they had identified the gene shared by the many members of an extensive Italian and Italian-American family who had Parkinson's,[2] it seemed inevitable that the gene responsible for the disease in almost everyone would be found. And that would lead to the discovery of the protein manufactured by the gene—and of drugs that could block the protein before it did its damage. Unfortunately, practically no one outside the one family appeared to share the gene discovered in 1996. Scientists soon located another gene that causes rare cases of Parkinson's in people under 20; this gene also turned up in some others who developed the disease much later in life. But for most of us, no genetic link has yet emerged. Instead, it may be that some complex combination of genes predisposes us to the disease if we come in contact with certain environmental poisons.

Of course, some progress has occurred. Researchers have learned more about the disease's basics: not yet its cause, but at least the mechanism by which it ravages certain brain cells. And they are developing new tools to help unlock Parkinson's secrets. Powerful imaging devices, which can peer inside the brain and see the disease's impact, may soon allow physicians to diagnose Parkinson's much more accurately than simply by observing patients' symptoms.

An accurate diagnosis is most valuable if it can be followed by effective treatment. And right now (in late 2001) there are probably more promising treatments on the horizon than at any time since levodopa became available. Researchers are hard at work on four techniques that show real promise of repairing or replacing Parkinson's dying nerve cells. If you asked two dozen neurologists to rank these four therapies in order of likelihood that they will one day offer substantial relief, you would probably get two dozen different answers. I outline here the leading clinical prospects as of 2001, with the replacement techniques first.

Fetal Tissue Transplants

Among tomorrow's treatments, fetal tissue transplants have undergone the most thorough testing. They have produced dramatic improvements in some patients, and at one point I considered fetal tissue transplants a likely course for me. But recent reports have proved discouraging, and the operation is all but impossible to get.

Swedish surgeons pioneered this approach in the 1980s by transplanting healthy dopamine-producing cells from aborted fetuses into the brains of people with Parkinson's. They discovered that the best target area for the new cells was not the substantia nigra, where the old cells were dying. You may remember that the substantia nigra's nerve cells deliver their dopamine to the nearby brain structure called the striatum. Newly transplanted fetal cells are too small to reach the striatum, and so surgeons figured out that they could inject the fetal cells right where the dopamine is needed—namely, the putamen, which is part of the striatum.

In the United States, fetal tissue transplants foundered on the politics of abortion, and Presidents Ronald Reagan and George Bush banned federal assistance for fetal tissue research from 1988 through 1993. For anyone who could afford the $40,000 fee or persuade an insurance company to pay, transplants were available at Good Samaritan Hospital in Los Angeles for a few years in the mid-1990s. Two neurosurgeons—I dubbed them "the cowboy and the communist"—operated with private research money. Dr. Deane B. (Skip) Jacques had put himself through the University of Colorado medical school by performing in rodeos; his partner, Dr. Oleg V. Kopyov, was a recent immigrant from Russia. When I spoke with them in 1997, they said they had performed more fetal tissue transplants than anyone outside Russia and Cuba. They were still developing their technique. They had determined, for example, that three was the ideal number of fetal donors: fewer than three did not yield enough cells, and more didn't seem to make any difference. They had not, however, satisfied themselves that they had found precisely the right place in the brain to inject the fetal cells.

The Parkinson's research community quietly condemned Jacques and Kopyov for exploiting patients' desperation by coaxing them into an operation that was very risky to the patients but lucrative to the surgeons. The Food and Drug Administration, which would have prohibited them from administering dangerous and untested drugs, has, strangely, no authority to police surgical procedures. But Jacques and Kopyov's patients—at least the two whose names they gave me— seemed satisfied with the results a year or two after their operations.

Jacques and Kopyov charted how sixty of their patients were faring a year after surgery and found that, on average, they had milder symptoms and were taking less medication than before. At the extremes, three patients dropped all anti-Parkinson's medications after the operation; three others showed no symptomatic improvement at all. Nine of the patients experienced negative effects, but for eight of these, the complications were blood clots and other problems that could have resulted from any kind of brain surgery. Only one patient suffered a transplant-related complication: severe dyskinesias. This condition was corrected in a second operation, a pallidotomy.[3]

Shortly after I talked with Jacques and Kopyov, their hospital shut down their program. Even before these surgeons started transplants, however, the operation had been tried elsewhere in the United States on a very small scale. The first patient was Don Nelson, and he offers living proof that fetal tissue transplants can work.

Don was only 32 years old in 1969 when the little finger of his left hand could no longer automatically strike the *a* key on his manual typewriter hard enough to make a mark. Because Don was so young, a series of mistaken diagnoses followed. An orthopedic surgeon blamed a damaged nerve in his left elbow and operated—to no avail. A neurosurgeon hypothesized a small tumor, so small he could not find it on a brain scan and so could not remove it. Finally, three years later, his left arm all but useless from stiffness and tremor, Nelson consulted Dr. Stuart Schneck, a University of Colorado neurologist, who quickly diagnosed Parkinson's. Levodopa temporarily controlled his symptoms, but within a few years, Don could no longer tolerate the pressure of his job as a corporate executive in the manufactured-housing industry. He resigned and bought a Tastee-Freez franchise, but that, too, soon became too stressful, and he quit working in 1980. His symptoms grew progressively worse—he needed a cane to walk without falling— and Dr. Schneck introduced him to a University of Colorado colleague, Dr. Curt Freed, who had overseen extensive fetal tissue transplant surgery on monkeys. With private funds donated by a Denver man whose brother had died with Parkinson's, Dr. Freed was ready to try his technique on humans. In a ten-hour operation that began late on November 8, 1988, and ended the next morning, the right side of Don's brain received about thirty thousand healthy cells from two fetuses.

Dr. Freed—a pharmacologist, not a surgeon—did not actually perform the operation. That was left to Dr. Robert Breeze, who was in his early 30s and looked even younger: so young that when he introduced himself to Don as his surgeon, Don instantly replied, "Oh no you're not." Yes he was, and the operation came off flawlessly. Don remained awake throughout and watched much of the surgery in the reflection on the glass door of a cabinet in front of him. Afterward, he found for the first time in nineteen years that his symptoms were diminishing. Within a year, he could do things around the house—painting and wallpapering a bedroom—that had been beyond him. After another couple of years, he had reduced his medication by about two-thirds and was still able to remodel two bathrooms and help his son put up drywall in his new house (tasks that no amount of surgery would enable me to do). But the operation had been performed only on the right side of Don's brain, and so it helped only the left side of his body. After three or four years, symptoms on the right side worsened. So in 1996, he received a second transplant of some sixty thousand fetal nerve cells on the left side of his brain. This time the surgeon drilled into his skull through the forehead rather than the back, and the surgical equipment attached to his head made it difficult for him to see. But he could feel. "I felt the drill go into the scalp, stop, and then pulled out," he wrote later. "Then came the needles, the first one the doctor counted slowly to 31, and the second to 39, just a bit deeper. I am sure the measurement was not in inches. I've been called a 'fathead,' but the distance from the back to the front of my head isn't 39 inches. Once the needles were in place, Dr. Freed pumped in the cells. The needles were extracted with sort of a scraped feeling as they came out. Dr. Breeze commented that maybe they need to use more WD-40 [motor oil] to lubricate them. At this point, about 34 minutes had passed."

"After six weeks I could tell I was getting better," Don told me four years after the second operation. "I had better use of my hands, and my walking and my speech were improved. Now I take four Sinemet 25/100s a day [about half as much levodopa as I take]. I can ride a bike, and in the summer of 1999 I drove all the way to Canada and Michigan. My wife, Carolyn, was with me, but I wouldn't let her drive. I can walk, but I freeze when I try to walk through a narrow passage. The doctors are working on that."

This is an undeniable success story. Thirty-one years into the disease—as I write this—Don is doing so well that he usually avoids Parkinson's support groups because he feels guilty about his good fortune. But one case proves little; even an operation that fails 99 percent of the time works one time in a hundred.

While George Bush was president through 1992, no government research money was available for a careful study of fetal tissue transplants. And even after President Bill Clinton lifted the ban on fetal tissue research in 1993, most researchers stayed away for fear that a new president might reimpose restrictions. Of the grant proposals received by the government, the NIH approved only two, one headed by Dr. Freed at the University of Colorado, the other by Dr. Warren Olanow at the Mount Sinai School of Medicine in New York. Both proposed to run clinical trials of fetal tissue transplants.

The two proposals were controversial. Surgeons planned to divide volunteers for their clinical trials into two groups of equal size. Those in one group would undergo operations to transplant fetal nerve cells into their brains. Those in the other (the control group) would also undergo operations, but nothing would be transplanted. None of the patients would be told whether their operation was the real thing or a sham. Many highly respected medical figures argued that sham surgery was unethical because it placed patients in considerable danger. Why would Parkinson's patients agree to participate in this study, knowing that they faced all the dangers of brain surgery but only a 50-50 chance of its potential advantages? Because they are desperate: a 50 percent chance of undergoing an operation that might cure them is better than a 100 percent chance of getting gradually worse. The justification for having a control group is the same as in the testing of new drugs. In drug trials, one group of participants is typically given sugar pills—the technical word is *placebos*—instead of the medication being tested. Researchers can't be sure that new treatments work unless they can compare their results with an identical, control group of patients who don't receive the experimental therapy. And unless both groups think they may be receiving the new treatment, they are not identical. Many people report that they feel better, at least for a while, if they take sugar pills that they think are the real medicine—the placebo effect. (In fact, my wife has the rare ability to cure a headache just by getting out a bottle of aspirin, without ever taking any.)

Dr. Freed's trial started first, in May of 1995. He collected forty volunteers, only twenty of whom received the real cells. The surgeons operated on both sides of the brain at once; bilateral transplants do not carry the same dangers as some other Parkinson's operations when performed on both sides. The patients were evaluated at regular intervals after their surgery at the Columbia-Presbyterian Medical Center in New York, where none of the examiners initially knew which patients had the transplants and which had the sham operations. A year after their operations, the patients were told whether they had had the real operation or the sham. The twenty patients who had not received fetal tissue were given the opportunity to have the real operation, and fourteen of them chose to have it. Nearly six years after the first operation, Dr. Freed and his colleagues reported on their findings.[4]

I interpreted the results as a mixture of promise and disappointment, although the *New York Times* prominently reported that the trial had proved fetal tissue transplants don't work. And two top officials of the National Institute of Neurological Disorders and Stroke, writing in the same issue of the *New England Journal of Medicine* in which Dr. Freed's paper was published, said even if transplants worked, they would be impractical. Assume, conservatively, that 10 percent of the Parkinson's population sought the operation and that only two fetuses were needed for each: that would require 200,000 fetuses. The two officials urged people like me not to be too greedy. "The brain is a most complex structure," they wrote, "so incremental results on the way to cures are to be welcomed rather than dismissed as less than perfect."[5]

In fact, Dr. Freed and his team wrote that the fetal tissue took hold and grew in seventeen of the twenty patients who initially received it. Autopsies showed thriving fetal tissue in the brains of two patients who died soon after their operations of unrelated causes—one when she had a heart attack, and one when she drove her car into a tree that had fallen across a highway during Hurricane Fran in 1996. But thriving fetal tissue did not always translate into milder symptoms. A year after their operation, the patients no older than 60 at the time of the operation seemed to a team of doctors to be better off than the control group. Their muscles and joints were not as rigid and they could move more quickly, although their tremors had not moderated. But the older patients showed no significant improvement. And when the patients themselves were asked whether they felt better than before the operation, the younger and older patients alike reported no change.

Still more interesting were the results after another two years. In the eyes of the doctors, the younger patients continued to improve, and the older ones began to. Ominously, however, five of the thirty-four patients who ultimately received fetal tissue developed debilitating dyskinesias—uncontrollable movements similar to those experienced by people with Parkinson's when they've taken too much levodopa or when their brains can no longer reliably convert the levodopa to dopamine. All five of these patients were 60 or younger at the time of their operation. Three of them had had the real operation the first time, and two had had the sham surgery first.

One of these individuals lives near me in suburban Maryland. Kassim Shehim, a native of Eritrea, came to the United States to study history in college and has been here ever since. Diagnosed with Parkinson's at the age of 38, in 1984, he had to abandon his teaching position at Idaho State University three years later. By the mid-1990s, he was having trouble walking. So he signed up for Dr. Freed's 1996 trial, believing it couldn't make matters worse, and he was in the group receiving transplants. "At first, I thought I had the placebo," he told me. "But after about three months, I started getting better." He could feel himself loosening up, and his ability to move greatly improved. The improvements stopped after about a year, but his dyskinesias didn't. When I visited him, he seemed almost symptom-free when he walked. But when he sat or lay down, he lost control of many of his muscles. His neck moved this way and that, causing his head to swing from side to side and front to back as if on a spring. Similarly, his arms moved in random patterns, and his speech was scarcely intelligible. So I talked with him as we walked around the block. He said he felt better off with the surgery than he had been before. He was planning another operation—this time deep brain stimulation—in hopes of taming the dyskinesias.

Another of those who developed what were regarded as severe dyskinesias was in New York's World Trade Center on September 11, 2001—and lived to tell about it. George Doeschner, an electrician who was 57 years old on that memorable date, had the sham surgery in 1996 and elected to have the real thing in January of 1999. His tremor improved, although he also began bobbing up and down when he walked —"dancing," as he described it. He was able to keep working, however, and on September 11, he was rewiring the thirty-fourth floor of the first of the two World Trade Center towers to be hit by a hijacked jetliner. Luckily, Doeschner is at his best in the morning. His "dancing" was not severe enough to prevent him from joining the parade of people who walked down the stairs to safety. He was able to keep up with the flow and was at a safe distance when the second tower was hit and both towers collapsed. He was back at work two days later, and when I caught up with him, he was working on a building in midtown Manhattan several miles away from the World Trade Center.

Some Parkinson's experts found the fate of the five patients who developed dyskinesias so serious that they recommended abandoning fetal tissue transplants altogether. Dr. Paul E. Greene of the Columbia University College of Physicians and Surgeons, one of the doctors who evaluated patients after their operations, called the uncontrollable movements "absolutely devastating."[6] Dr. Freed, by contrast, said the answer might be as simple as injecting fewer fetal cells and adjusting the site where they are injected. It also remains possible that the second NIH-funded trial of fetal tissue transplants, which uses different kinds and amounts of fetal cells, will yield more promising results.

Even if scientists were to perfect fetal tissue transplants, tissue of just the right age and blood type would not always be available when and where it was needed. And even if it were, the politics of abortion might place the procedure off-limits in the United States. The passions have split brother from brother and father from son. Former Rep. Michael Bilirakis, chairman of a key health subcommittee in the House of Representatives in the 1990s, opposed fetal tissue research even though his own younger brother's death had been accelerated by Parkinson's.[7] The father of an acquaintance of mine who had a fetal cell transplant refused to talk to his son for months afterward. But as I see it, fetal tissue research doesn't encourage women to have abortions. Clinton's executive order permitting fetal tissue research prohibited rewarding women for contributing the aborted fetus to science. In fact, they could not be told they could donate the fetus until after the abortion. Even zealous anti-abortion advocates could not find a case of an abortion motivated by the prospect of donating the fetus. Yet the extreme abhorrence of abortion continues to make fetal tissue research a risky specialty. This is where stem cells come in.

Stem Cells

At the end of 1998, research teams led by James Thomson at the University of Wisconsin and John Gearhart at the Johns Hopkins University found, almost simultaneously, what may prove to be an alternative to fetal tissue. Working with human embryos and fetuses, the researchers found cells that, in the proper chemical environment, could be both reproduced in unlimited quantities and transformed into almost any kind of cell. This ability to produce limitless supplies of any kind of cell seemed almost too good to be true. The possibilities are vast: cells for the pancreas that could enable diabetics to produce insulin again; kidney cells for people who would otherwise need dialysis; dopamine-producing cells for those of us with Parkinson's. And new embryos or fetuses would not have to be collected to meet new demand for stem cells. Researchers would merely look inside their laboratory refrigerators and tap their stocks of self-reproducing stem cells.

Of course, medical science isn't this simple. Researchers must still learn how to transport stem cells to the place in the body where they're needed. And the understanding of how to convert stem cells into the cells of different organs is still primitive: it wouldn't do to inject stem cells into the brain if they grew into a hand or a gallbladder. But the progress over just a few years has been astonishing. At the NIH, Dr. Ron McKay and his collaborators first determined how to generate unlimited quantities of dopamine-producing neurons from mouse stem cells.[8] Then they did the same with human stem cells—using the resulting cells to repair rat brains that had been intentionally damaged. Researchers believe they can find the chemical triggers that make stem cells generate dopamine-producing nerve cells. Perversely, it might be harder to stop the process than to start it. In this nightmare, stem cells run wild inside the brain, causing a kind of cancer.

Stem cells hold many advantages over fetal tissue. For starters, scientists can make the supply; they don't have to wait for an aborted fetus with the right blood type. Likewise, they can be sure of exactly what cell line the cells came from. Stem cells can be found in the excess frozen embryos in fertility clinics. These tiny fertilized eggs were generated for couples unable to have children the usual way; the woman's eggs were fertilized by the man's sperm in a laboratory dish. The result was many more fertilized eggs than couples wanted. The clinics froze the extras— estimated at a hundred thousand in all—and have already begun discarding them.

Even these embryonic stem cells outrage many anti-abortionists. To them, an embryo is a life, and no one has a right to end it. Zealots from this camp lined the road to Dr. Gearhart's laboratory in Baltimore after his success in isolating stem cells, carrying signs reading, "Gearhart and Johns Hopkins, Nazi Partners in Eugenic Experimentation." But others in the pro-life camp reach a different conclusion. Sen. Gordon Smith of Oregon, whose mother was a first cousin to the late Rep. Mo Udall, finds it humane to treat diseases with embryos that would otherwise be discarded. "Part of my pro-life ethic is to make life better for the living," he has said.[9] In the mid-1990s, Congress placed a moratorium on the use of human embryos for research purposes. Only in 1999 did the NIH interpret the law to allow publicly funded research if the stem cells came from fertility clinics' excess embryos and not from embryos created exclusively to provide cells for research.

Two years later, President George W. Bush further limited federally funded stem cell research by restricting it to cell lines already in existence on August 9, 2001, the day that he announced his policy. Research was permissible, Bush said, if no additional embryos had to be destroyed. But no federal money would support research with embryos destroyed after August 9. The president and his top aides said some sixty cell lines already existed, enough, they said, to realize stem cells' potential for curing disease. Many researchers were not so sure. They said that some of the cell lines were not suitable for research and that others were privately owned and would not be made available.

Bush hoped that a way out of this ethical dilemma would be provided by "adult" stem cells. Some researchers have reported that they can grow stem cells in laboratory dishes without using human embryos or fetuses. In one experiment, researchers extracted some cells from human bone marrow and mixed them in a dish with just the right chemical triggers—and the bone marrow cells grew into nerve cells.[10] In two others, bone marrow cells from adult mice produced nerve cells when injected into the brains of other mice.[11] These experiments raised the possibility that doctors could simply use a long needle to extract some of my bone marrow and use it to grow dopamine-producing brain cells. This would eliminate not only the ethical dilemma but also the danger that my immune system would reject cells that had originated in a different body. As I write, however, it's still unknown whether adult stem cells are vibrant and versatile enough to perform the demanding job of growing new brain cells.

If not, there are two other promising experimental therapies that try to make the most of the nerve cells that have survived Parkinson's. Both these therapies strive to protect nerve cells that are still healthy and reinvigorate those that are dying.

GDNF

One chemical under investigation is a hormone with a name so long— glial cell line–derived neurotrophic factor—that it is almost always abbreviated: GDNF. Fittingly, the molecule is so big that it can't cross the blood-brain barrier. That, for people with degenerative brain diseases, is a pity, because GDNF seems to protect living nerve cells and restore dying ones. GDNF was all the rage in the early 1990s, when Amgen, a California biotech company, tried to convert it into a therapeutically useful form. Amgen ran a test that involved injecting the hormone directly into the brain. The test failed. The hormone apparently never reached the part of the brain (the substantia nigra) where it was needed.

Now genetic engineering may be coming to the rescue. A team of researchers led by Dr. Jeffrey Kordower, a pharmacologist at Chicago's Rush Presbyterian–St. Luke's Hospital, have grafted GDNF's genetic material onto a virus, which they then injected into the substantia nigra of five rhesus monkeys that had been given Parkinson's symptoms.[12] There the viruses did what ordinarily makes viruses so dangerous: they inserted their own genes into the cells of the host animals. But in this case, the genes carried by the viruses directed the manufacture of GDNF. In three of the five monkeys, the GDNF so increased the supply of dopamine that the monkeys became symptom-free. One of the other monkeys died, and the other was not helped.[13] I don't like those odds: a 60 percent chance of a cure but a 20 percent chance of dying. Of course, scientists will now try to improve the odds, and they may succeed. Will they be able to work fast enough to help me? Shortly after the experiment was completed in 2000, Dr. Kordower said that clinical trials in humans might still be three to five years away. A year later he was much more optimistic. I talked with him when he was in Washington to receive a research grant of half a million dollars from the local Washington chapter of the National Parkinson Foundation, which found his research the most promising in the nation. At that time he thought human trials might be able to begin in less than a year. But even if they do, researchers will still need time to determine the proper amount of GDNF-virus to deliver and the ideal place to deliver it. So it figures to be years before the government approves gene therapy. That's why scientists are looking hard for a smaller molecule—one that can cross the blood-brain barrier—to repair the substantia nigra. They might just have found one.

Immunophilins

When my Parkinson's was diagnosed, no one had a clue that a drug designed to turn off the body's immune system might be a key to arresting or even reversing Parkinson's disease. In early 2001, such a drug was undergoing trials in humans. Its discovery demonstrates the value of basic scientific research. It provides a cautionary tale for those who insist that society pay only for research promising a quick payoff. Dr. Ted Dawson, a Johns Hopkins neurologist, belongs to the team whose research led to the drug. When I asked him how the team did it, he said, "We sort of stumbled upon it. Our general idea was correct, but our original hypothesis was wrong. But we kept following the leads we uncovered until we got to where we are today."

First they investigated a class of proteins called immunophilins that help turn off the body's immune system. Immunophilins became important in the 1950s, when the first kidney and liver transplants forced doctors to find ways to prevent the host (recipient) body's immune system from rejecting a foreign organ. Surgeons developed drugs that, when they interacted with the body's immunophilins, blocked the immune system and let the transplanted organs take hold.

Until the early 1990s, scientists did not know how the immune-suppressing drugs worked. Then in 1991, researchers at Harvard identified the protein (calcineurin) in the immune system that was rendered inactive by the transplant drugs. That finding caught the eye of the Hopkins team, which had already observed that the brain had large concentrations of immunophilins. The Hopkins team was sure the high concentrations were no accident. "We figured they must be doing something important," Dr. Joe Steiner, another team member, recalled. "Nature wouldn't let that happen without a good reason."

What was the reason? Answering that question took many years of hard work. It led to a remarkable discovery: the transplant drugs might also protect many brain cells from damage—and possibly even help them grow. The problem was that these drugs also immobilized the immune system: anyone regularly using them could die from a random infection. The trick was to modify one of these drugs so that it would still promote neuron growth yet not disarm the immune system. Over the next several years, the research team devised a number of derivatives that accomplished this feat. By then, Steiner was working for a small Baltimore biotech company called Guilford Pharmaceuticals. Guilford patented the compounds and licensed production to Amgen, which had the resources to bring a new drug to market. The FDA authorized clinical trials for the first of the experimental drugs (AMG 474-00) beginning late in 2000.[14] Three hundred recently diagnosed Parkinson's patients were given either AMG 474-00 or a placebo for six months.

The results were discouraging. By some measures, those who took

AMG 474-00 were worse off after six months than was the control group. Altogether, the experimental group fared no better and no worse at the end of the trial than the control group. But this won't be the last we hear from the immunophilins. AMG 474-00 was only the first of several such compounds patented by Guilford and licensed to Amgen. Of course, none of them may perform any better than the first. Even before the disappointing results with AMG 474-00, many scientists were wary. If the immunophilins actually protected nerve cells while helping them grow, no one knew the mechanism. And Amgen's earlier failure with GDNF had not been forgotten. But the immunophilins have one huge advantage over GDNF—they are small enough to cross the blood-brain barrier. This means they can be taken as pills rather than injected directly into the brain. For me and those like me, time is short. I hope that if any of the immunophilins make it to market, my substantia nigra will still have enough surviving dopamine cells to rejuvenate.

It will be my good fortune if any of these potential cures materializes. If that happens, my debt will be not only to scientists but also to all those Parkinson's activists who have lobbied for more research. They could just as easily have taken my path: trying to live with Parkinson's pretty much as before. Instead, they chose the more stressful route of confronting the nation's medical and political establishments and demanding a crash effort to find a cure. They are people like Perry Cohen, my fellow Washingtonian, who became involved practically the moment he was diagnosed, and Jim Cordy, the Pittsburgh activist who made a 180-degree switch from hiding his Parkinson's to becoming an outspoken advocate. In these ranks, no one has done more than Joan Samuelson.

Joan, a California lawyer, was 37 when diagnosed with Parkinson's in 1987. As I did three years later, she assumed that medical science would find a cure or at least an improved treatment that would help her. Unlike me, she took no medication, fearing that it would damage the baby she was trying to conceive. By the early 1990s she couldn't get around without a cane or a wheelchair. At about that time, she read reports that Swedish surgeons had successfully transplanted fetal nerve cells into the brains of Parkinson's patients. She was appalled to discover that in the United States, Presidents Reagan and Bush had banned the use of federal money for such research at the insistence of anti-abortion forces.

Joan contacted the national Parkinson's groups to see what they were doing about the research ban. Their responses stunned her: the American Parkinson Disease Association didn't support lifting the ban; the

National Parkinson Foundation wasn't interested in the issue; the United Parkinson's Foundation didn't get involved in politics; and the Parkinson's Disease Foundation was studying the matter. So Joan looked for a sympathetic member of Congress. She found one in Rep. Henry A. Waxman, the Los Angeles Democrat who chaired one of the House health subcommittees. As it happened, Waxman's subcommittee was putting together a hearing on the fetal tissue research ban, and it invited Joan to testify. She appeared with Anne Udall, the daughter of the congressman, and Dr. Curt Freed, the University of Colorado expert on fetal tissue transplants.

Washington intrigued Joan. Her marriage was breaking up—she never did get pregnant—and she abandoned her law practice. Her condition had improved when she began taking levodopa, and she started her own, highly political Parkinson's organization. The national Parkinson's groups, which hardly ever agreed on anything, unanimously urged her not to. They didn't know Joan. Their opposition only encouraged her. At the end of 1992, she launched the Parkinson's Action Network.

"I was acting out of self-preservation," she told me. "Research money was flowing to other diseases but not to Parkinson's." She compares her devotion to political action to my decision to write this book: a form of denial, a way of concentrating on the present to avoid thinking about the future. "My way of dealing with a crisis is to try to take control of it," she said, "to make myself the boss."

On his second full day in office in 1993, President Clinton overturned the ban on the use of federal funds to conduct fetal tissue research. Joan formed a highly effective alliance with the second generation of Udalls—which now includes two members of Congress—and PAN quickly became the Parkinson's community's most effective voice in Washington. In 2001, thirteen years into her disease, Joan still looked great and could speak before large audiences without betraying any signs of stress. Clearly, her medications (she also cites ample amounts of acupuncture, yoga, and psychiatric counseling) deserve some of the credit. But she knows the day is approaching when the disease will overwhelm today's pills. If medical science is ready with something better, she will have herself to thank—and, possibly, the actor Michael J. Fox.

In 1999, Fox added his celebrity power to the Parkinson's cause by acknowledging that he had had the disease for seven years and demanding that the medical community work for a cure. Famous yet self-effacing, a glamorous star yet a dedicated family man, Fox is the perfect poster child for Parkinson's disease, as effective as Christopher Reeve, of Superman fame, for spinal cord injury. Fox's public appearances before Congress may have lacked some of the drama of Reeve's. After breaking his neck in a horse-riding accident, Reeve needed a ventilator just to breathe. But as Fox twisted from side to side in committee witness chairs, his condition was apparent for everyone to see. Congressional office doors that had opened only a crack for other Parkinson's advocates flew wide open for Fox. The new Michael J. Fox Foundation for Parkinson's Research quickly became a dominant force nationally in raising both government and private money to find a cure.

Waiting for a cure is growing more frustrating as my symptoms mount. Must the scientific process be so agonizingly slow? Can't researchers cut some corners? Does the government have to be so conservative in deciding which drugs get to market? The deck is so stacked against finding a cure. None of the potential therapies on the horizon in 2001 gets at the root cause of Parkinson's or the mechanism by which it systematically attacks the brain's dopamine-producing cells. And for good reason: the cause and the mechanism remain mysteries. As long as they do, developing a cure will be something of a shot in the dark. Mihael Polymeropoulos, who led the research team that discovered the first Parkinson's gene, told me: "Finding the cure from where we are now is like getting on a horse and trying to ride to the nearest star. In order to have a treatment or a cure, you have to know what you're dealing with. I consider understanding the mechanism of a disease to be the *sine qua non* of treatment."

Even better than curing Parkinson's would be stopping it before it develops. By the time symptoms appear, as many as 80 percent of the cells of the substantia nigra are already dead. What if doctors could spot a substantia nigra in which, say, only 60 percent of the cells were dead? And what if they could stop the deterioration right there? The answer is that nobody would develop Parkinson's. But these are two huge "ifs," and progress is slow. On the first, scientists are developing ever more sensitive machines that use subatomic particles to "see" inside the brain: they can detect one of the proteins involved in delivering dopamine from its home nerve cell into the synapse.[15] Because these contraptions are fabulously expensive, they can't be used to check everyone. But if researchers could consult the genes to tell who was predisposed to Parkinson's, they could then screen the people most at risk. And if family histories yielded the identities of persons most likely to have positive results on genetic tests, the initial genetic screening could be limited to this group. Of course, discovering incipient Parkinson's is worthless if the disease can't be headed off. Researchers are also searching hard for ways to protect the brain from whatever kills the cells of the substantia nigra. That's the holy grail of Parkinson's research. Only when it is found will Parkinson's be truly conquered.

Epilogue: *Light in the Darkness*

> Science allows mystery but not magic, strangeness beyond wild imagining
> but no spells of witchery, no cheap and easy miracles.
> —Richard Dawkins, *Unweaving the Rainbow*

HERE ARE SOME RECENT MOMENTS in a life with Parkinson's.

July 23, 2000, 11 A.M.; room 304, St. Joseph's Hospital, Baltimore. This is simple joy. I'm holding Evelyn tight. She can't express herself very well—she is only ten hours old—but then, neither can I. Her beauty, and her very existence, overwhelm me. Theresa Nicol, Judy's daughter, is bouncing around on the bed, exhausted by twenty-one hours of labor but too excited to rest. Her husband, Edward Herskovits, is getting her a bagel, her first food in a day and a half. Evelyn Leah Herskovits is Theresa and Eddie's first child—and Judy's first grandchild. I am thrilled. Evelyn may not have my genes, but her mother has absorbed a lot of my upbringing. That's good enough for me: she's my granddaughter too.

Same day, 12 hours later; somewhere between Baltimore and Washington on Interstate 95. Now comes the pain. While Judy heads home in one car, the three kids and I are driving back to Washington in the other. Anne is at the wheel; after a big dinner, all I can do is shake and sweat. Luckily, Anne can concentrate on the road no matter how high the volume on the Beatles tape, although once or twice I warn her to slow down to 70. My leg muscles defy all efforts to relieve their tension. I move my legs up and down from the floor to the glove compartment, much like walking. They remain stiff and painful. I tuck them under me on the seat. That doesn't help either. I'm sweating as if running a marathon in the Amazon rain forest. When we arrive home ninety minutes later, I'm drained. It's exhausting to stay stiff for that long and sweat so much. My undershirt is drenched. It feels as if somebody just fished it out of a lake.

In our eleven-year relationship, Parkinson's disease has earned my deep respect. It is more sinister than an infection that can be killed with antibiotics, more mysterious than the runaway cell growth of cancer.

153

Although it was first identified nearly two hundred years ago, medical researchers have still not solved many of its puzzles. What causes it? Why does it kill some brain cells but not others? What is the mechanism of destruction? The brain jealously guards its secrets.

Parkinson's creeps up when you least expect it; takes over your life so slowly that you scarcely notice it; frustrates every defense with which you try to stop it. When you think you have it under control on one front, it opens another. Levodopa has stopped your tremor? Just wait: the side effects will get worse. Think you can live with the physical symptoms? That's when the disease assaults your mind.

Physically compensating for each new disability is hard enough. Adjusting mentally is harder. After living for many years as an independent adult and planning to continue doing so for many more, you have to accept your newfound status of dependence. At the same time, you must resist the temptation to believe your disabilities make you less than human. You can't let it bother you when perfect strangers stare at you as you lurch down the street, when sales clerks wonder why you can't fish a dollar bill from your wallet. Most difficult of all, you have to cope with the knowledge that, unless a cure suddenly emerges, you face a future more challenging than the present. And all this you have to do even as the disease depletes the very energy you need to fight back.

Cunning and insidious, Parkinson's is intent on taking over my very existence. I spend much of each day thinking about it and coping with it. It is becoming my obsession, the embodiment of evil: what Moby Dick was to Captain Ahab; what Professor Moriarty was to Sherlock Holmes. This, I now realize, is exactly what I dreaded in my early years with the disease. Then I was repelled by accounts of others' meticulous medication schedules. Now I wear an alarm watch that vibrates every three hours to remind me to take more pills. Then I regarded support group members as "them." Now I think of them as "us."

For both Captain Ahab and Sherlock Holmes, the object of their obsession became the agent of their destruction. Ahab dies when he harpoons the great white whale but the rope coils around his neck and yanks him into the sea. Holmes at least manages to take Moriarty with him when he plunges to his death at Reichenbach Falls. Will Parkinson's twist its rope around my neck? Will it push me over the edge of the falls?

Next day; home. Agitated after returning from Baltimore, I sleep fitfully. I awaken at 2 A.M. but manage to get back to sleep. I repeat the cycle at

2:45. But when I wake up again at 3:30, my legs won't settle down. Still trying to sleep—and unwilling to risk waking Judy—I move to the couch downstairs. After a futile half hour, I give up. I lie on the floor for my three minutes of daily stretching exercises and four swayback push-ups. Then I head for the bathroom. I can't shave—my legs are too wobbly, and I can't make the razor find my face. Violating my rule not to resort to pills before 5:30 or 6 o'clock, I take four kinds all at once. Then I search for things to do while waiting for the pills to work. The only way I can read is to move enough that I stop shaking. So for the better part of an hour I read the previous day's newspaper while walking round and round the kitchen, like a sheepdog circling a small herd. For another hour I wash, sort, and freeze several quarts of blackberries that Judy and Margaret picked the day before on the way to Baltimore. Still I am too shaky to shave. It is as if I had never taken the first round of pills. So I take my second round at the hour when I prefer to take my first. Then I shower and, with the medication now helping, manage a crude job of shaving. That's how the day keeps going. Pills every three hours don't quite keep up. At 10 A.M., when I drive Margaret to an orthodontist appointment, I have to stop the car on the way and walk around for a few minutes to alleviate my tremor. Back home, I concentrate enough to write for half an hour. But by 3 P.M., I have already taken five rounds of pills; just a week earlier, that would have got me through an entire day.

What's going on? Have I lost serious new ground to the disease? I don't think so. For my eleven years with Parkinson's, it has progressed in a pattern. The symptoms get much worse for a day or two, usually in response to outside stress. Then they subside to where they were before. At that point they worsen almost imperceptibly until some new source of stress causes another temporary spike in my symptoms. Meanwhile, a new medication might emerge to improve my condition. When I switched to a new dopamine agonist three years ago, I cut back my usual daily dose of levodopa from six pills to five. The disease erased that gain. Entacapone, which I began taking a year or two later, restored it—temporarily. Now I'm just about where I was before I switched to the new dopamine agonist. The disease moves with a glacier's speed—and power. Every new kind of pill is a warm summer that creates the illusion of gains. But each summer is followed by a winter when the glacier resumes its relentless advance.

This I accept as my fate—another of Parkinson's lessons. In tenth grade, Margaret read *Oedipus the King*, Sophocles' great tragedy. The story is familiar: Oedipus, his mother, and his father come to unspeakable grief (Oedipus kills his father and marries his mother) by trying to escape what the gods had preordained. At first, I denied my fate. Now, thanks largely to preparing this book, I accept it for what it is—a life on the downward slide. What I don't accept is this: that such a life is no life at all. To accept that would be to quit living.

Parkinson's wins if it makes me focus on the long term—and give up. My strategy is to concentrate on the short term—and keep going. I set challenging short-term goals (finishing each chapter of this book provided a dozen of them) and strive to achieve them. I think not about my future but about Anne's, Margaret's, William's, and now little Evelyn's. Their future is my future. Their healthy bodies are my body. I live to enjoy their living.

Judy and the children are blessings far more powerful than Parkinson's curse. Judy is the family's genuine intellectual, always learning, always teaching. She let me defy the odds and have a family—and not just any family. I think often of Anne's spending a weekend with me in Philadelphia to close down my aunt and uncle's apartment after they had moved to a nursing home. I told her then that I could always count on her when I really needed her—and I still can. I think of Margaret's English teacher's words on a report card: "She is taking significant responsibility for her own learning, and clearly that puts her in capable hands." I think of Will's stealing the show in his school's production of *Pajama Game*. I pranced through the crowd during intermission as if holding up a sign that said, "Father of the star."

I leave no great professional achievements. My works, as surely as those of Ozymandias, will be lost. What I can contribute to posterity are my children—and, I fervently hope, their children and theirs and theirs, for as long as there is a human race.

What if I had no children, no Judy?

What kind of a burden will I place on them if I become incapacitated for a long period of time but refuse to die? My family has done well at caring for its old. While my own parents dodged that duty, others in the family filled in. Uncle Bruce, my mother's younger brother, never married, and when his mother gradually grew feeble, Bruce cared for her in his apartment for her final several years. Now Bruce is on the receiving end. In his 80s, he has difficulty walking, the result of diseased veins in his legs. He lives alone in an apartment in downtown St. Louis, the town of his birth. Though only a few blocks from where his beloved Cardinals play baseball, Bruce is too lame to go there. In fact, he can't get to the grocery store or the doctor's office on his own. There to help him is our family angel, my mother's cousin. Five years older than Bruce, Ethel Ellersiek is losing only a little of her spunk. Single all her life, she took care of her father, incapacitated for many years by a stroke, and then her mother, who declined gradually until her death in the 1970s.

Unless Ethel is fortunate enough to drop dead suddenly, as my mother did, even she will one day need care—and there will be no Ethel to give it. Judy and I are ready to fill that role. Our basement infirmary is empty, Judy's mother having moved out in 1999. Caring for Ethel the way she has cared for so many others—it's the least we can do. How unfair it would be to subject her to the cold inhumanity of a nursing home after all she has done to provide warm, human care to so many others.

Parkinson's makes me likely to spend more time on the receiving end than the giving end of Ethel's equation. Eleven years since my diagnosis, I'm still surprisingly self-sufficient. I have to prepare for the possibility that in another eleven, I might be hopelessly dependent. What if I'm helpless by the time I'm 65, and live to be 80? Judy says she would keep me out of an institution at all cost. I suspect that would be the children's first instinct as well. I hope they will reconsider. I don't want any of my family to sacrifice their best years for my worst.

Maybe they won't have to. In my eleven years with Parkinson's, new treatments have become available that promise to extend the good years with Parkinson's. I already use two of the new drugs: pramipexole, an improved dopamine agonist; and entacapone, a COMT inhibitor. And surgery can suppress Parkinson's symptoms after the pills no longer can. If I had to choose a form of surgery today, it would be deep brain stimulation. This is the one operation that is reversible, and it can be done safely on both sides of the brain. Because I can still manage pretty well on pills alone, I'm not ready to undergo the ordeal of brain surgery. But I can imagine myself one day with electrodes in my brain and a magnet-controlled pacemaker under my collarbone.

If I'm really lucky, even deep brain stimulation will not be necessary. It seems increasingly likely that today's research will deliver tomorrow's cure. It might involve chemicals that find their way to the scene of the damage and repair the broken nerve cells. It might involve replacing dead or diseased brain cells with vigorous cells removed from aborted fetuses or generated by human stem cells. It might even be a form of therapy still unknown to the general public. Parkinson's research is bursting. For the first time since my diagnosis, there is reason to believe that we will soon have the means to slow, stop, or even reverse Parkinson's relentless progress. Will it be soon enough for me? That is a question no one can answer. Merely posing it requires peering into the dark future—something that all of us with Parkinson's have trained ourselves not to do.

I prefer to dwell on what the disease has meant to me in its first eleven years. Like all formidable adversaries, it has been a good teacher. It has taught that the human spirit does not easily succumb. I have lots of company. Millions of people in all corners of the globe are waging the same battle against this ailment and scores of other degenerative diseases and disabilities. In their number are powerful politicians and hard-working factory hands, famous entertainers and ordinary parents. Given one life to live, they live it as best they can.

Parkinson's has given me new respect for the human mind. I have come to admire the brain's infinite complexity, to respect all it can do and to forgive it for what it cannot. I regard it with the same sense of awe that I feel when I look up at the sky on a clear night and behold the vast expanse of the universe.

And it has infused in me a deep appreciation of family. Of my parents, for the values they left me. Of Judy, for the love (and the children) she has given me. And of the children, for embodying a hopeful future.

Admiration for humanity. Reverence for nature. Love of family. These are my core beliefs. These are my religion. This I have learned from my disease. Parkinson's, do your worst. You can't rob me of that.

Glossary

L-AAAD. The enzyme that acts as the catalyst in converting levodopa to dopamine in the bloodstream and the brain. Its full name is L-aromatic amino acid decarboxylase.

Amantadine. An antiviral drug found to alleviate Parkinson's symptoms, especially in the early stages of the disease. Its brand name is Symmetrel.

Amino acid. Any of the chemicals that are the building blocks of proteins.

Anticholinergic. Any drug that inhibits the release of acetylcholine, one of the brain's neurotransmitters.

Artane. A common anticholinergic drug. Its generic name is trihexyphenidyl.

Basal ganglia. The masses of nerve cells located deep in the cerebrum, including the putamen and the caudate nucleus (which together make up the striatum) and the globus pallidus.

Blood-brain barrier. The "wall" within blood vessels that blocks many large molecules in the bloodstream from passing into the brain.

Bradykinesia. Slowness of movement, one of the cardinal features of Parkinson's disease.

Brainstem. The part of the brain near the connection with the spinal cord, consisting of all the parts of the brain except the cerebrum and cerebellum.

Bromocriptine. One of the dopamine agonists. Its brand name is Parlodel.

Capillary. The narrowest of the blood vessels.

Carbidopa. A drug that prevents the transformation of levodopa into dopamine. It is the other ingredient, in addition to levodopa, in Sinemet. Because it does not cross the blood-brain barrier, it protects levodopa only in the bloodstream and not in the brain.

Catalyst. A compound that is necessary for a particular chemical reaction to take place but emerges from the reaction unchanged.

CAT scan. Computerized axial tomography scan: a scan using X-rays to provide a cross-sectional view of the brain or other body part. Also called a CT (computed tomography) scan.

Caudate nucleus. A component of the brain's basal ganglia. The caudate nucleus and the putamen constitute the striatum, a part of the brain immediately downstream from the substantia nigra.

Cerebellum. A part of the brain, under the cerebrum, that controls voluntary muscle movement.

Cerebrum. The thinking part of the brain and, in humans, the biggest part, extending around the outside of the brain.

Cogwheel rigidity. Stiffness of a limb in which, if force is applied to bend the limb, the joint reacts with cogwheel-like jerks. This is often a sign of Parkinson's disease.

COMT. Catechol-O-methyltransferase: an enzyme that breaks down levodopa and dopamine.

Comtan. A medication that blocks the action of COMT in the bloodstream, thereby allowing more levodopa to reach the brain. Its generic name is entacapone.

Control group. In a research study, a group of individuals who resemble in every aspect except one a group receiving a medication or undergoing a medical procedure. Members of the control group may be taking a placebo instead of the medication being tested, or they may lack a particular condition shared by the test group, such as Parkinson's disease.

Deep brain stimulation. An operation in which electrodes that can deliver an electrical current are implanted in one of several parts of the brain—the thalamus, the globus pallidus, or the subthalamic nucleus. A wire running under the skin of the neck connects the electrodes to a battery-powered pacemaker implanted under the collarbone. A magnet passed over the pacemaker can adjust the electrical current or turn it off, as needed. The current short-circuits electrical pathways where the electrodes are implanted.

Dopamine. One of the neurotransmitters that carry messages across synapses from one nerve cell to another. Dopamine is manufactured in the nerve cells of the substantia nigra. A shortage of dopamine prevents the proper messages from reaching the striatum, resulting in the movement abnormalities that characterize Parkinson's disease.

Dopamine agonist. One of several drugs, very close in structure to dopamine, that work directly on some of the dopamine receptors in the striatum. The receptors behave as if they had come in contact with dopamine itself.

Dyskinesia. Involuntary, abnormal movement. In Parkinson's, this usually takes the form of writhing, twisting motions.

Dystonia. A state of abnormally contracted or relaxed muscles, frequently causing cramps.

Eldepryl. A medication that prevents the enzyme MAO-B from breaking down dopamine in the brain. Its generic name is selegiline.

Entacapone. A medication that blocks the action of the enzyme COMT in the bloodstream. Its brand name is Comtan.

Enzyme. A protein that acts as a catalyst, enabling chemical reactions to occur without itself being changed.

Essential tremor. A rapid tremor, usually of the hands and arms when they are in use but sometimes of the head and voice. It often, but not always, runs in families. It is also known as familial tremor.

FDA. Food and Drug Administration: the federal agency that approves drugs before they can go on the market.

GDNF. Glial cell line–derived neurotrophic factor: one of a group of proteins that promote and sustain the growth of nerve cells.

Glial cell. An electrically inactive brain cell that provides physical support for the neurons, or nerve cells.

Globus pallidus. A component of the brain's basal ganglia. The globus pallidus lies just downstream from the striatum.

Growth factor. A chemical produced by the body that regulates growth of cells and tissues.

Hormone. A chemical manufactured in one part of the body and carried by the bloodstream to do a job in another part of the body.

Hypomimia. An expressionless face, a symptom of Parkinson's disease.

Hypophonia. A soft and often monotone voice, a frequent symptom of Parkinson's disease.

Immunophilin. A protein that helps turn off the body's immune system.

Ion. An atom or group of atoms carrying an electrical charge.

Levodopa. The chemical that is converted into dopamine by the enzyme L-AAAD in the bloodstream and the brain. It is the intermediate product of the two-stage chemical reaction that converts the amino acid tyrosine into dopamine in the brain. It is also known as L-dopa.

MAO-B. Monoamine oxidase-B: an enzyme that breaks down dopamine into its waste products.

Micrographia. Extremely small handwriting—a common Parkinson's symptom.

Midbrain. The uppermost portion of the brainstem, containing the substantia nigra.

Mirapex. One of the dopamine agonists. Its generic name is pramipexole.

MRI. Magnetic resonance imaging: an extremely powerful tool for looking at structures inside the body using magnetism instead of X-rays.

Neuron. A nerve cell carrying an electrical current that enables it to communicate with other neurons.

Neurotransmitter. A chemical messenger that transmits electrical impulses across the synapses.

NIH. National Institutes of Health: the government agency responsible for much of the nation's biomedical research.

On-off fluctuations. In persons with Parkinson's, the sudden progression from being steady to being symptomatic: from being "on" medication to being "off."

Orthostatic hypotension. Low blood pressure upon standing after sitting or lying down, causing dizziness, light-headedness, and sometimes fainting. It can be a symptom of Parkinson's disease or a side effect of the medication.

Pallidotomy. An operation in which a part of the globus pallidus is destroyed. In Parkinson's disease, part of the globus pallidus is overactive, and a pallidotomy is designed to restore it to the proper level of activity.

Parkinsonism. A group of related diseases marked by tremor and movement difficulties. Parkinson's disease is the most common; others include progressive supranuclear palsy and multi-system atrophy.

Parlodel. One of the dopamine agonists. Its generic name is bromocriptine.

Pergolide. One of the dopamine agonists. Its brand name is Permax.

Permax. One of the dopamine agonists. Its generic name is pergolide.

Placebo. A sugar pill administered to some participants in a drug test. Because those in the test do not know whether they are taking the real medication or a placebo, their expectations do not color their response to the pills.

Pramipexole. One of the dopamine agonists. It is sold under the brand name Mirapex.

Putamen. A component of the brain's basal ganglia. The putamen, along with the caudate nucleus, constitutes the striatum. Neural circuits passing through first the substantia nigra and then the putamen govern body movement.

Requip. One of the dopamine agonists. Its generic name is ropinirole.

Ropinirole. One of the dopamine agonists. It is sold under the brand name Requip.

Selegiline. A medication that blocks MAO-B from attacking dopamine in the brain. Its brand name is Eldepryl.

Sinemet. Medication containing levodopa and carbidopa.

Stem cell. A cell that, depending on its chemical environment, can grow into almost any kind of cell in the body.

Stereotactic surgery. Brain surgery in which the skull is bolted to a frame to keep it perfectly still.

Striatum. A section of the brain's basal ganglia. The striatum consists of two primary parts, the putamen and the caudate nucleus. It receives information from the parts of the brain responsible for thinking and for collecting information from the sense organs. It processes this information and sends the results to the globus pallidus.

Substantia nigra. A part of the midbrain that manufactures the neurotransmitter dopamine; so named because it contains a black pigment. In a healthy brain, the dopamine transmits information to the striatum. In Parkinson's disease, most of the substantia nigra cells are degenerating, and there is not enough dopamine to communicate with the striatum.

Subthalamic nucleus. A collection of nerve cells deep in the brain that have intimate connections with the substantia nigra and the basal ganglia. It is overactive in Parkinson's disease.

Symmetrel. An antiviral medicine found to alleviate the symptoms of Parkinson's disease. Its generic name is amantadine.

Synapse. The tiny gap between nerve cells in the brain (and elsewhere in the nervous system).

Tasmar. A medication that blocks the action of COMT (the enzyme that breaks down levodopa) in the bloodstream. Its generic name is tolcapone.

Thalamotomy. An operation in which cells in a specific part of the thalamus are destroyed.

Thalamus. A large, egg-shaped collection of nerve cells. It is connected to the basal ganglia.

Tolcapone. A medication that inhibits the action of COMT. Its brand name is Tasmar.

Trephination. A Stone Age–era surgery in which a hole was drilled in the head to let out demons thought to be causing disease and to relieve the pressure thought to be responsible for headaches.

Tyrosine. An amino acid, found in most proteins. In the presence of the proper enzymes in the substantia nigra, tyrosine is converted first into levodopa and then into dopamine. In Parkinson's disease, the brain has an ample amount of the enzyme necessary to transform levodopa into dopamine, but not enough of the enzyme that first transforms tyrosine into levodopa.

Tyrosine hydroxylase. The enzyme that acts as the catalyst in converting tyrosine into levodopa.

Notes

INTRODUCTION: AS I LAY TREMBLING

James Parkinson, *An Essay on the Shaking Palsy* (London: Whittingham and Rowland, for Sherwood, Neely, and Jones, 1817), p. ii.

1. Richard Restak, *Brainscapes* (New York: Hyperion, 1995), p. 28.

CHAPTER 1: DENIAL AND IGNORANCE

Parkinson, *Shaking Palsy*, p. 3.

1. Although I did not find it at the time, Parkinson himself offered a particularly vivid description of one of his end-stage patients: "As the debility increases and the influence of the will over the muscles fades away, the tremulous agitation becomes more vehement. It now seldom leaves him for a moment; but even when exhausted nature seizes a small portion of sleep, the motion becomes so violent as not only to shake the bed-hangings, but even the floor and sashes of the room. The chin is now almost immoveably bent down upon the sternum. The slops with which he is attempted to be fed, with the saliva, are continually trickling from the mouth. The power of articulation is lost. The urine and faeces are passed involuntarily; and at the last, constant sleepiness, with slight delirium, and other marks of extreme exhaustion, announce the wished-for release." *Shaking Palsy*, pp. 8–9.

2. Parkinson believed the source of the shaking palsy was not the brain but the spinal cord. He recommended the following treatment: "blood should first be taken from the upper part of the neck, unless contraindicated by any particular circumstance. After which vesicatories should be applied to the same part, and a purulent discharge obtained by appropriate use of the Sabine Liniment, having recourse to the application of a fresh blister, when from the diminution of the discharging surface, pus is not secreted in a sufficient quantity." *Shaking Palsy*, pp. 58–59.

3. Paul Starr, *The Social Transformation of American Medicine* (New York: Basic Books, 1982), p. 55.

4. Gustavo C. Roman, Zhen-Sin Zhang, and Jonas H. Ellenberg, "The Neuroepidemiology of Parkinson's Disease," in *Etiology of Parkinson's Disease*, ed. Jonas H. Ellenberg, William C. Koller, and J. William Langston (New York: Marcel Dekker, 1995), p. 203.

5.   Roger Duvoisin, "History of Parkinsonism," *Pharmacology and Therapeutics* 32, no. 1 (1987), pp. 1–17.

6.   For example, W. R. Gowers, practicing as a London physician eighty years after Parkinson, put his money on the cerebral cortex, the outer surface of the brain, which is now known to carry out the brain's loftiest functions. W. R. Gowers, *Diseases of the Nervous System*, vol. II (London: J. & A. Churchill, 1893), p. 651.

7.   Jean-Martin Charcot, *Lectures on the Diseases of the Nervous System*, trans. George Sigerson (Philadelphia: Henry C. Lea, 1879), pp. 120, 124.

8.   Frederick Peterson, "Paralysis Agitans," in *Familiar Forms of Nervous Diseases*, ed. M. Allen Starr (New York: William Wood, 1890).

9.   L. Ordenstein, *Sur la paralysie agitante* (Paris: A. Delahaye, 1868), p. 25.

10.   Gowers, *Diseases of the Nervous System*, p. 637.

11.   Lawrence I. Golbe, "Genetics of Parkinson's Disease," in Ellenberg, Koller, and Langston, *Etiology*, pp. 122–124.

12.   Matthew A. Menza et al., "Dopamine-Related Personality Traits in Parkinson's Disease," *Neurology* 43 (Mar. 1993), pp. 505–508.

13.   National Parkinson Foundation, www.parkinson.org.

14.   Golbe, of the Robert Wood Johnson Medical School in New Brunswick, N.J., cites four studies of identical twins in which at least one twin had Parkinson's. Both identical twins had the disease in only five cases, not statistically different from the three cases out of sixty-six in control groups of fraternal twins. Lawrence I. Golbe, "Genetics of Parkinson's Disease," in Ellenberg, Koller, and Langston, *Etiology*, p. 120.

CHAPTER 2: MYSELF BEFORE PARKINSON'S

Louis E. Bisch, "Turn Your Sickness into an Asset," *Reader's Digest*, Nov. 1937.

1.   Richard Dawkins, *The Selfish Gene* (Bungay, Suffolk, U.K.: Oxford University Press, 1989), p. 19.

CHAPTER 3: THE MAGNIFICENT BRAIN

Emerson Pugh, c. 1938, as quoted by his son, George E. Pugh, in *The Biological Origin of Human Values* (New York: Basic Books, 1977), p. 154.

1.   It turns out that I'm not the only one who finds writing to be therapeutic. A recent study of patients with two other chronic

diseases—asthma and arthritis—found that those who wrote about
their conditions were not only psychologically but also physically bet-
ter off than those who did not. See Joshua M. Smyth, Arthur A.
Stone, Adam Hurewitz, and Alan Kaell, "Effects of Writing about
Stressful Experiences on Symptom Reduction in Patients with
Asthma or Rheumatoid Arthritis," *Journal of the American Medical
Association* 281, no. 14 (Apr. 14, 1999), pp. 1304–1329.

2.   The two enzymes are commonly known by their acronyms: *MAO-B,*
      for *monoamine oxidase,* and *COMT,* for *catechol-O-methyltransferase.*

3.   It may seem inefficient for predators to kill dopamine practically as fast
      as the brain can manufacture it. But in fact, the dopamine cycle is an
      ingenious system for ensuring that the body has just enough of the
      chemical. Left alone, dopamine would eventually wear out from over-
      use. Without a constant fresh supply, there would very soon be none
      of it at all. And with a steady stream of new dopamine and no way to
      rid the brain of the old, a serious glut would develop.

4.   Dr. Lucien Cote of Columbia Presbyterian Medical Center in New
      York is among those who think that Parkinson's disease causes people
      not to smoke or to quit smoking because smoking's rewards depend
      on a good supply of dopamine. In Parkinson's, the dopamine supply
      falls below the reward level long before it causes tremors and the other
      symptoms. See Lucien Cote, "Depression: Impact and Management
      by the Patient and Family," *Neurology* 52, suppl. 3 (Apr. 1999), pp.
      S7–S9. For a good survey of the confusion, see Anne-Maria Kuopio et
      al., "Environmental Risk Factors in Parkinson's Disease," *Movement
      Disorders* 14, no. 6 (1999), pp. 928–939.

5.   It seems only fitting that the evidence of a link between mercury and
      Parkinson's is ambiguous. Dr. Abraham Lieberman, medical director
      of the National Parkinson Foundation, reported in a recent letter to the
      Wall Street Journal (of all places) that the disease is no more common
      among people who handle mercury professionally—dentists, makers
      of dental amalgams, mercury miners, and mercury processors—than it
      is among the rest of the population. Neurological disorders resulting
      from mercury contamination, Dr. Lieberman wrote, are quite distinct
      from Parkinson's disease. Abraham Lieberman, "Mercury Isn't a
      Cause of Parkinson Disease," *Wall Street Journal,* May 31, 2001, p.
      A-17.
          That doesn't seem to square with the findings of researchers who
      compared fifty-four Parkinson's patients in Singapore with a ninety-
      five-member control group. They found that, as a group, the Parkin-

son's patients had considerably higher mercury levels in their blood than the control group. C. H. Ngim and G. Devathasan, "Epidemiological Study on the Association between Body Burden Mercury Level and Idiopathic Parkinson's Disease," *Neuroepidemiology* 8, no. 3 (1989), pp. 128–141.

6. Prime among the chemicals thought to play a role in destroying the nerve cells are oxidizing agents that readily destroy vital components of living cells. Hydrogen peroxide is an example of a particularly potent oxidizing agent. In looking within the cells, researchers are focusing on the mitochondria, the structures that generate the energy that keeps cells active, as the place where the damage occurs.

7. M. C. de Rijk et al., "Prevalence of Parkinsonism and Parkinson's Disease in Europe: The Europarkinson Collaborative Study," *Journal of Neurology, Neurosurgery, and Psychiatry* 62, no. 1 (1997), pp. 10–15.

CHAPTER 4: ESCAPING ABROAD
Charles Caleb Colton (1780–1832).

1. Professor Marsden died in the United States early in 1999 while working as a visiting researcher at the National Institutes of Health.

2. U.S. Census Bureau, Report No. P60-211 (Washington, D.C.: Government Printing Office, Sept. 28, 2000).

3. The pills I took consisted of 250 milligrams of levodopa, the chief ingredient, plus 25 milligrams of carbidopa, which is a kind of bodyguard that enables the levodopa to travel in the bloodstream from the intestine to the brain without being broken down into useless components.

4. The comments by McCurdy's bosses come from affidavits in Larry's equal employment opportunity grievance, filed with the Health and Human Services Department.

CHAPTER 5: THE DARKEST HOUR
Ernst Wynder quoted in the *New York Times,* Sept. 30, 1975.

1. Stephen S. Rosenfeld, *The Time of Their Dying* (New York: W. W. Norton, 1977).

2. David McCullough, *Truman* (New York: Simon & Schuster, 1992), pp. 983–988.

3. Russell S. Phillips, Mary Beth Hamel, Kenneth E. Covinsky, and Joanne Lynn (eds.), Supplement to the *Journal of the American Geriatrics Society* 48, no. 5 (May 2000). See particularly Ellen P. McCarthy

et al., "Dying with Cancer," p. S110; and Emese Somogyi-Zalud et al.,
"Elderly Persons' Last Six Months of Life," p. S131.

4. Denise Grady, "At Life's End, Many Patients Are Denied Peaceful
Passing," *New York Times*, May 29, 2000, p. A1.

5. For the Sicilian study, see Letterio Morganente et al., "Parkinson Disease Survival," *Archives of Neurology* 57 (Apr. 2000), pp. 507–513. For
earlier studies, see, for example, E. C. Louis, K. Marder, L. Cote, M.
Tang, and R. Mayeux, "Mortality from Parkinson's Disease," *Archives
of Neurology* 54, no. 3 (Mar. 1997), pp. 260–264. "Levodopa therapy
for Parkinson disease has improved the quality of life," they write,
"but mortality rates remain high." Likewise, a study of all Parkinson's
patients from Minnesota's Olmsted County who were seen at the
Mayo Clinic from 1964 to 1978 found that even for those who began
levodopa therapy early in the course of their treatment, death rates exceeded those of the general population. R. J. Uitti, J. E. Ahlskog, D.
M. Maraganore, M. D. Muenter, E. J. Atkinson, R. H. Cha, and P. C.
O'Brien, "Levodopa Therapy and Survival in Idiopathic Parkinson's
Disease," *Neurology* 43, no. 10 (Oct. 1993), pp. 1918–1926.

6. Abraham Lieberman, www.parkinson.org/survive.htm.

7. Sidney Dorros, *Parkinson's: A Patient's View* (Washington, D.C.:
Seven Locks Press, 1989).

CHAPTER 6: TODAY'S DRUGS

Plutarch, "Demetrius," in *Lives*, trans. John Dryden, rev. Arthur Hugh
Clough (New York: Modern Library, Random House, 1932), p. 1073.

1. Oleh Hornykiewicz, "From Dopamine to Parkinson's Disease: A Personal Research Record," in *The Neurosciences: Paths of Discovery,* ed.
Frederick E. Samson and George Adelman (Cambridge, Mass.:
Birkhauser Boston, 1992), p. 130.

2. The Latin prefix *levo* means "left." There is also a D-dopa (the Latin
word *dexter* means "right"). This has exactly the same component
atoms joined together in the same way but configured as the mirror
image to L-dopa, just as two gloves in a pair are the mirror image of
each other. The configuration matters: D-dopa is chemically inactive,
whereas L-dopa is anything but.

3. Arvid Carlsson, Margit Lindqvist, and Tor Magnussen, "3,4-
Dihydroxyphenylalanine and 5-Hydroxytryptophan as Reserpine Agonists," *Nature* 180 (Nov. 30, 1957), p. 1200.

4. No one knew it at the time, but Birkmayer had quite a sordid past. He

signed up for Hitler's SS in 1938 and served for a year before the SS discovered that, although Birkmayer didn't know it, he was part Jewish. He was promptly drummed out of the SS. See Harold L. Klawans, "The Second Belling of the Cat," *MD*, Sept. 1991, pp. 89–92.

5. Walther Birkmayer and Oleh Hornykiewicz, "Der L-3,4-Dioxyphenylalanin (= DOPA)—Effekt bei der Parkinson-Akinese," *Wien Klin. Wochenschr.* 73 (1961), pp. 787–788.

6. George C. Cotzias, "Metabolic Modification of Some Neurologic Disorders," *Journal of the American Medical Association* 210 (Nov. 17, 1969), pp. 1255–1262.

7. Besides entacapone, the other medication that attacks COMT is tolcapone (brand name Tasmar). I tried tolcapone first, but it seemed to have no effect. And at about that time, it was implicated in the death from liver failure of at least two Parkinson's patients. So I dropped tolcapone and later started taking entacapone. As of this writing, no further deaths from tolcapone have been reported since new regulations took hold requiring strict monitoring of liver function.

8. The drugs are Sinemet ($2.47, for two and a half pills a day at 99 cents per pill), Mirapex ($5.52, for three pills a day at $1.84 per pill), Comtan ($8.05, for five pills a day at $1.61 per pill), and generic versions of selegiline (81 cents for a single pill per day) and Artane (trihexyphenidyl) (9 cents for half a pill per day). It's interesting that the addition of Comtan to my potpourri saved me about half a Sinemet per day, or about 50 cents. But the five Comtans that I had to take added $8.05 to the daily bill. (All prices as of early 2001.)

9. For a particularly well-documented case, see David Willman, "The Rise and Fall of the Killer Drug Rezulin," *Los Angeles Times*, June 4, 2000, p. A-1.

10. For a case study involving a medication for high blood pressure and prostate enlargement, see Sheryl Gay Stolberg and Jeff Gerth, "How Companies Stall Generics and Keep Themselves Healthy," *New York Times*, July 23, 2000, p. 1.

11. A generic version of Sinemet is also available, and I've tried it twice. Maybe it's all in my head, but both times the generic seemed substantially inferior to the real thing. Dr. Reich says a small share of his patients—about one in twenty or thirty—respond as I do. My insurance company, waiving its usual practice, reimburses me for the full cost of the brand-name drug.

12. Some forms of psychosis are linked to an excess of dopamine in parts

of the brain other than the substantia nigra. Medication containing levodopa becomes the raw material for more dopamine not only in the substantia nigra, where it is needed, but also in parts of the brain where it is harmful. Likewise, drugs that suppress dopamine where it is harmful also tend to suppress it in the substantia nigra.

CHAPTER 7: TODAY'S SURGERIES

Dr. John Kirklin quoted in *Time* magazine, May 3, 1963.

1. W. J. Bishop, *The Early History of Surgery* (London: Robert Hale, 1960), pp. 20–23.

2. The choice of terms was controversial. Horsley and Clarke used the phrase *stereotaxic surgery*, derived from the Greek words for "three-dimensional" and "arrangement." Gradually that evolved to *stereotactic*, with the Latin word for "touch" forming the second half of the word. Classics purists objected to mixing Greek and Latin, but others thought that "touching" came closer to what they were doing than "arranging." The practitioners of the new art voted in 1973 to call themselves the World Society for Stereotactic and Functional Neurosurgery.

3. Mark Hallett and Irene Litvan, "Evaluation of Surgery for Parkinson's Disease," *Neurology* 53 (Dec. 1999), pp. 1910–1921.

4. Nina King, "Parkinson's: A Long, Strange Trip; Why One Woman Let a Swedish Surgeon Burn out a Portion of Her Brain," *Washington Post*, Nov. 3, 1998, p. Z-12.

5. Mark S. Baron et al., "Treatment of Advanced Parkinson's Disease by Unilateral Posterior Gpi Pallidotomy: 4-Year Results of a Pilot Study," *Movement Disorders* 15, no. 2 (Mar. 2000), pp. 230–238.

6. Jennifer Fine et al., "Long-Term Follow-up of Unilateral Pallidotomy in Advanced Parkinson's Disease," *New England Journal of Medicine* 342, no. 23 (June 8, 2000), pp. 1708–1714.

7. A compilation of studies found thalamotomy to be at least moderately effective against tremor in 79 to 85 percent of cases, compared with 50 to 60 percent for pallidotomy. See Hallett and Litvan, "Evaluation of Surgery."

8. Researchers in the Netherlands found thalamic stimulation to be the equal of thalamotomy in relieving tremor—and with fewer bad side effects. P. Richard Schuurman et al., "A Comparison of Continuous Thalamic Stimulation and Thalamotomy for Suppression of Severe Tremor," *New England Journal of Medicine* 342, no. 7 (Feb. 17, 2000), pp. 461–468.

9.   J. A. Obeso, et al., "Deep-Brain Stimulation of the Subthalamic Nucleus or the Pars Interna of the Globus Pallidus in Parkinson's Disease," *New England Journal of Medicine* 345, no. 13 (Sept. 27, 2001), pp. 956–963.

10.   P. Limousin et al., "Electrical Stimulation of the Subthalamic Nucleus in Parkinson's Disease," *New England Journal of Medicine* 339, no. 16 (1998), pp. 1105–1111.

11.   Unpublished figures from the National Center for Health Statistics.

12.   G. Selby, "Stereotactic Surgery," in *Handbook of Parkinson's Disease*, ed. W. C. Koller (New York: Marcel Dekker, 1987), pp. 421–435.

CHAPTER 8: AN INSIDIOUS BEAST
Parkinson, *Shaking Palsy*, pp. 4–5.

1.   My stiff right arm probably accounted for the "frozen shoulder" I developed just as Dr. Reich was diagnosing me. I could scarcely elevate my right arm to the horizontal position, much less raise it over my head—a common consequence of rigid arm muscles. I still exercise my arms every morning to prevent a recurrence.

2.   National Parkinson Foundation, www.parkinson.org/impotenc.htm.

3.   See, for instance, William J. Weiner, Lisa M. Shulman, and Anthony E. Lang, *Parkinson's Disease: A Complete Guide for Patients and Their Families* (Baltimore: Johns Hopkins University Press, 2001).

4.   Elise Tandberg, Jan P. Larsen, and Karen Karlsen, "Excessive Daytime Sleepiness and Sleep Benefit in Parkinson's Disease: A Community-Based Study," *Movement Disorders* 14, no. 6 (June 1999), pp. 922–927.

5.   Jo-anne Marr, "The Experience of Living with Parkinson's Disease," *Journal of Neuroscience Nursing* 23, no. 5 (Oct. 1991), pp. 325–329.

6.   Meryl Brod, Gerald A. Mendelsohn, and Brent Roberts, "Patients' Experiences of Parkinson's Disease," *Journal of Gerontology* 53B, no. 4 (1998), pp. 213–222. The complete list is revealing:

Writing	93%	Rigidity	72
Extra physical effort	82	Posture	72
Awkward, clumsy	81	Tremor	69
Rising from chair	81	Drug side effects	69
Forgetful	80	Slowing of thinking	68
Walking	78	Nervousness	68
Lack of energy	78	Being understood	65
Dressing, grooming	75	Sleeping	62

Feelings of depression	61	Bathing/showering	42
Falling	61	Meeting others' expectations	40
Driving	59	Feeding self	38
Drooling	58	Feeling of social isolation	37
Confusion	57	Reading	34
Dependence on others	52	Unable to work	33
Meeting family responsibilities	50	Sexual activity	33
Feelings of being a burden	50	Boredom	32
Concentrating	48	Toileting	32
Making decisions	48	Keeping self-respect	26
Expressing feelings	47	Being taken seriously	24
Swallowing	44		

7. C. Warren Olanow and Jose A. Obeso, "Preventing Levodopa-Induced Dyskinesias," *Annals of Neurology* 47, suppl. 1 (Apr. 2000), pp. S167–S174.
8. See Y. Agid, "Levodopa: Is Toxicity a Myth?" *Neurology* 50, no. 4 (Apr. 1998), pp. 858–863.
9. M. G. Murer et al., "Chronic Levodopa Is Not Toxic for Remaining Dopamine Neurons, but Instead Promotes Their Recovery, in Rats with Moderate Nigrostriatal Lesions," *Annals of Neurology* 43, no. 5 (May 1998), pp. 561–575.
10. Y. Agid, T. Chase, and D. Marsden, "Adverse Reactions to Levodopa: Drug Toxicity or Progression of Disease?" *Lancet* 351 (Mar. 21, 1998), pp. 851–852.
11. See, for example, G. Fabbrini et al., "Motor Fluctuations in Parkinson's Disease: Central Pathophysiological Mechanisms, Part I," *Annals of Neurology* 24, no. 3 (Sept. 1988), pp. 36–71.
12. Parkinson Study Group, "Pramipexole vs. Levodopa as Initial Treatment for Parkinson's Disease: A Randomized, Controlled Trial," *Journal of the American Medical Association* 284, no. 15 (Oct. 18, 2000), pp. 1931–1938; O. Rascol, D. J. Brooks, A. D. Korczyn, et al., "A Five-Year Study of the Incidence of Dyskinesia in Patients with Early Parkinson's Disease Who Were Treated with Ropinirole or Levodopa," *New England Journal of Medicine* 342 (2000), pp. 1484–1491; J. S. Rakshi et al., "Is Ropinirole, a Selective D2 Receptor Agonist, Neuroprotective in Early Parkinson's Disease?" *Neurology* 50, suppl. 4 (1998), p. A330.
13. Y. Agid et al., "Levodopa in the Treatment of Parkinson's Disease: A Consensus Meeting," *Movement Disorders* 14, no. 6 (1999), pp. 911–

913. The three American dissenters were Warren Olanow, Stanley Fahn, and Gerald Cohen.

14.   William J. Weiner, "Is Levodopa Toxic?" *Archives of Neurology* 57 (Mar. 2000), pp. 408–410.

15.   S. Frucht et al., "Falling Asleep at the Wheel: Motor Vehicle Mishaps in Persons Taking Pramipexole and Ropinirole," *Neurology* 52, no. 9 (June 10, 1999), pp. 1908–1910.

16.   For some of the critics, see *Neurology* 54, no. 1 (Jan. 11, 2000), pp. 274–277.

17.   What actually happened that morning was a little more complicated. Because her days were eventful and difficult, Joan had taken a time-released Sinemet tablet at bedtime the night before to help her sleep. It worked so well—and she set the alarm so early—that she was perfectly steady when she woke up. She told the camera crew (from ABC's *20/20*) not to worry; soon she would be her usual incapacitated, nearly paralyzed self. After nearly an hour, she was finally in bad enough shape to crawl into bed and "wake up" a second time. (The show aired on October 11, 1999.)

18.   So uncertain are the estimates of Parkinson's patients with depression that the American Parkinson Disease Association uses two quite different guesses in the same publication. Its handbook for those who develop the disease at an early age estimates a 50 to 75 percent incidence early in the text but only a 40 percent incidence toward the end.

19.   A team of Finnish researchers found that depression, more than any other Parkinson's symptom, eroded patients' quality of life. Anne-Maria Kuopio et al., "The Quality of Life in Parkinson's Disease," *Movement Disorders* 15, no. 2 (2000), pp. 216–223.

20.   Abraham Lieberman, "Dementia in Parkinson's Disease," www.parkinson.org/pddement.htm.

21.   T. A. Hughes, "A 10-year Study of the Incidence of and Factors Predicting Dementia in Parkinson's Disease," *Neurology* 54 (2000), pp. 1596–1692.

22.   Lieberman, "Dementia in Parkinson's Disease."

23.   Francis J. Pirozzolo et al., "Cognitive Impairments Associated with Parkinson's Disease and Other Movement Disorders," in *Parkinson's Disease and Movement Disorders*, 2d ed., ed. Joseph Jankovic and Eduardo Tolosa (Baltimore: Williams & Wilkins, 1993), pp. 491–501.

24.   William J. Weiner, Alireza Minagar, and Lisa M. Shulman, "Quetiapine for L-Dopa-Induced Psychosis in PD," *Neurology* 54, no. 7 (Apr. 11, 2000), p. 1538.

25.   Stephen G. Reich, "Parkinson's Disease and Related Disorders," in
       Kelley's Textbook of Internal Medicine, 4th ed., ed. H. David Humes
       (Baltimore: Lippincott Williams & Wilkins, 2000).
26.   The Parkinson's Action Network merged early in 2000 into the new
       Michael J. Fox Foundation for Parkinson's Research, but the marriage
       didn't last: the two organizations soon had their separate identities, al-
       though they continued to work closely together.
27.   John C. Rogers, Testimony to the Subcommittee on Defense of the
       House Appropriations Committee, March 29, 2000.

CHAPTER 9: KEEPING THE BEAST AT BAY

       Adelle Davis, *Let's Eat Right to Keep Fit,* rev. ed. (New York: Harcourt
       Brace Jovanovich, 1970).
1.   Susan B. Levin (senior ed.), *Coping with Parkinson's Disease,* 2d ed.
       (St. Louis: American Parkinson Disease Association, n.d.), pp. 53, 73.
       The first edition was published in 1986.
2.   For my money, the best all-purpose physician-written guidebooks are
       Parkinson's Disease: A Complete Guide for Patients and Families, by
       Drs. William J. Weiner and Lisa M. Shulman of the University of
       Maryland, Baltimore, and Dr. Anthony E. Lang of the University of
       Toronto; and *Parkinson's Disease: A Guide for Patient and Family,*
       4th ed. (New York: Raven Press, 1996), by Drs. Roger C. Duvoisin
       and Jacob I. Sage. The ideal bedroom is described in an American
       Parkinson Disease Association handbook called "Be Independent!"
       by Marilyn B. Robinson, a registered nurse. The National Parkinson
       Foundation, which is in the final stages of publishing its own com-
       prehensive guide to dealing with Parkinson's, already has a website
       full of information (www.parkinson.org).
3.   This observation on the importance of remaining active is neither
       deeply insightful nor original. See, for example, Leslie D. Frazier,
       "Coping with Disease-Related Stressors in Parkinson's Disease,"
       Gerontologist 40, no. 1 (2000), pp. 53–63; and Jacqui Handley, "Psy-
       chological Aspects of Parkinson's Disease," *Elder Care* 11, no. 4 (June
       1999), pp. 34–36.
4.   Lucien Cote, "Depression: Impact and Management by the Patient
       and Family," *Neurology* 52, suppl. 3 (Apr. 1999), pp. S7–S9. Cote is
       not the only expert who feels this way. For those who find Parkinson's
       has made their life's goals unreachable, Danish researcher Svend An-
       dersen advises adjusting the goals rather than simply giving up: "Small
       achievements can result in attaining control over part of life once

again." Svend Andersen, "Patient Perspective and Self-help," *Neurology* 52, suppl. 3 (Apr. 1999), pp. S2–S28.

5.   Pam R. Rajendran, Richard E. Thompson, and Stephen G. Reich, "The Use of Alternative Therapies by Patients with Parkinson's Disease," *Neurology* 54, suppl. 3 (Apr. 2000), pp. A471–A472.

6.   L. M. Shulman et al., "Acupuncture Therapy for the Symptoms of Parkinson's Disease," *Movement Disorders* 15, suppl. 3 (2000), p. 113.

7.   Stephen J. Birch and Robert L. Felt, *Understanding Acupuncture* (Edinburgh: Churchill Livingston, 1999).

8.   Chris McGonigle, *Surviving Your Spouse's Chronic Illness* (New York: Henry Holt, 1999), p. 4.

9.   J. H. Ellgring, "Depression, Psychosis, and Dementia," *Neurology* 52, suppl. 3 (Apr. 1999), pp. S17–S20.

10.   Morton Kondracke, *Saving Milly: Love, Politics, and Parkinson's Disease* (New York: Public Affairs, 2001).

11.   Susan Hamburger, Caregiver's Corner, www.parkinson.org.

12.   Dorros, *Parkinson's.*

CHAPTER 10: TOMORROW'S REMEDIES

Hippocrates, c. 400 B.C., from *The Aphorisms of Hippocrates, Prince of Physicians* (London: Humphrey Mosely, 1655), sect. I, aph. 6, p. 5.

1.   The legislation was named the Udall Bill after Rep. Morris K. Udall, who at the time was comatose as a result of a fall down the stairs, probably because of Parkinson's-related balance problems. It authorized the National Institutes of Health to spend an extra $100 million over the next five years to support Parkinson's research. In the years immediately before the Udall Bill, the NIH spent about $25 million to $30 million a year on Parkinson's research, or about $25 to $30 for every American with the disease. By contrast, the NIH spent about $100 on heart disease, $300 on cancer, and $1,000 on AIDS for each person with those diseases.

2.   Mihael H. Polymeropoulos et al., "Mapping of a Gene for Parkinson's Disease to Chromosome 4q21-q23," *Science* 274 (Nov. 15, 1996), pp. 1197–1199.

3.   D. B. Jacques, O. V. Kopyov, et al., "Outcomes and Complications of Fetal Tissue Transplantation in Parkinson's Disease," *Stereotactic and Functional Neurosurgery* 72, no. 2–4 (1999), pp. 219–224.

4.   Curt Freed et al., "Transplantation of Embryonic Dopamine Neurons for Severe Parkinson's Disease," *New England Journal of Medicine* 344, no. 10 (Mar. 8, 2001), pp. 710–719.

5. Gerald D. Fischbach and Guy M. McKhann, "Cell Therapy for Parkinson's Disease," *New England Journal of Medicine* 344, no. 10 (Mar. 8, 2001), pp. 761–763.

6. Paul Greene quoted in Gina Kolata, "Parkinson's Research Is Set Back by Failure of Fetal Cell Implants," *New York Times*, Mar. 8, 2001, p. A1.

7. I heard Bilirakis mention his brother publicly only once, at a hearing of his subcommittee on March 9, 2000. After referring to his brother's fate, he said, "The unborn little babies are also victims."

8. Sang-Hun Lee, Ron D. McKay, et al., "Efficient Generation of Midbrain and Hindbrain Neurons from Mouse Embryonic Stem Cells," *Nature Biotechnology* 18 (June 2000), pp. 675–679.

9. Gordon Smith quoted in the op-ed column in the *New York Times*, Nov. 1, 2000, p. A-31.

10. Dale Woodbury et al., "Adult Rat and Human Bone Marrow Stromal Cells Differentiate into Neurons," *Journal of Neuroscience Research* 61 (2000), pp. 364–370.

11. E. Mezey et al., "Turning Blood into Brain: Cells Bearing Neuronal Antigens Generated in Vivo from Bone Marrow," *Science* 290 (Dec. 1, 2000), pp. 1779–1782; T. R. Brazelton et al., "From Marrow to Brain: Expression of Neuronal Phenotypes in Adult Mice from Adult Bone Marrow-Derived Cells," *Science* 290 (Dec. 1, 2000), pp. 1775–1779.

12. Parkinson's disease can be induced in laboratory animals (and people, for that matter) by an overdose of the drug MPTP. The drug's dramatic impact was discovered when it turned up as an impurity in a batch of artificial heroin made in Los Angeles in the 1970s. Its story is told by Dr. William Langston in *The Case of the Frozen Addicts* (New York: Pantheon Books, 1995).

13. Jeffrey H. Kordower et al. "Neurodegeneration Prevented by Lentiviral Vector Delivery of GDNF in Primate Models of Parkinson's Disease," *Science* 290 (Oct. 27, 2000), pp. 767–773.

14. Technically, AMG 474–00 is not an immunophilin at all. It is a derivative of a drug that, when delivered to the body, joins forces with the immunophilins to immobilize the immune system: that makes it an immunophilin ligand—a compound that links up with the immunophilins. But for simplicity's sake, this category of potential anti-Parkinson's medication has come to be known as immunophilins.

15. Parkinson Study Group (Kenneth Marek et al.), "A Multicenter Assessment of Dopamine Transporter Imaging with DOPASCAN/SPECT in Parkinsonism," *Neurology* 55 (Nov. 2000), pp. 1540–1547.

Epilogue: Light in the Darkness

Richard Dawkins, *Unweaving the Rainbow: Science, Delusion, and the Appetite for Wonder* (Boston: Houghton Mifflin, 1998).

Index

Page numbers in italics refer to illustrations.